Strategic Analysis *for* Healthcare

Strategic Analysis *for* Healthcare

CONCEPTS AND PRACTICAL APPLICATIONS

Michael S. Wayland
Warren G. McDonald

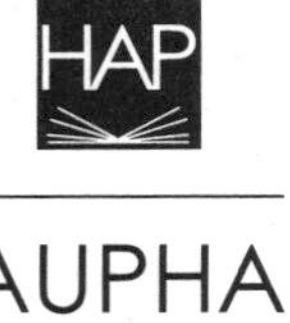

AUPHA
Health Administration Press, Chicago, Illinois
Association of University Programs in Health Administration, Arlington, Virginia

Your board, staff, or clients may also benefit from this book's insight. For more information on quantity discounts, contact the Health Administration Press Marketing Manager at (312) 424-9470.

20 19 18 5 4 3 2

Library of Congress Cataloging-in-Publication Data

Wayland, Michael S.
Strategic analysis for healthcare : concepts and practical applications / Michael S. Wayland and Warren G. McDonald.
pages cm
ISBN 978-1-56793-751-0 (alk. paper)
1. Health services administration. 2. Strategic planning. I. McDonald, Warren G. II. Title.
RA971.M23 2016
362.1068--dc23
2015026988

The paper used in this publication meets the minimum requirements of American National Standard for Information Sciences—Permanence of Paper for Printed Library Materials, ANSI Z39.48-1984. ♾™

Acquisitions editor: Tulie O'Connor; Project manager: Michael Noren; Cover designer: Brad Norr; Layout: Virginia Byrne

Found an error or a typo? We want to know! Please e-mail it to hapbooks@ache.org, and put "Book Error" in the subject line.

Health Administration Press
A division of the Foundation of the American College of Healthcare Executives
One North Franklin Street, Suite 1700
Chicago, IL 60606-3529
(312) 424-2800

Association of University Programs in Health Administration
2000 North 14th Street
Suite 780
Arlington, VA 22201
(703) 894-0940

This book is dedicated to our wives and families who support us, our friends who encourage us, and our professional colleagues at Methodist University, and across the globe, who inspire us.

CONTENTS

PREFACE

Organizational efforts to meet the challenges of the seemingly never-ending changes in contemporary healthcare require effective strategic analysis. We have to manage organizations operationally, but if we expect to survive in this ever-evolving healthcare marketplace, we also must focus on the future—and that is what strategic analysis is all about. Using sound analysis, organizations can develop strategies to help them not only survive, but also thrive, well into the future. Unfortunately, organizations often lack understanding on just how to accomplish that task effectively and efficiently.

This book presents a straightforward approach to the development of strategy for healthcare organizations. The clear explanations of specific concepts, the supporting examples, and the applied exercises approach the topic from both theoretical and practical perspectives, covering each individual method in an easy-to-read yet informative manner. The "toolbox" presented here contains more than just the typical SWOT analyses (though we do cover those extensively); it includes a wide variety of techniques sure to be useful in learning about the importance of strategy and how to develop it.

Contents of the Book

The book consists of 26 chapters, and from the very beginning to the final chapter, it addresses strategy development in a practical and straightforward fashion. The book is designed to aid both the professor in teaching the material and the students as they seek to improve their understanding of the strategic management process. The content evolved from notes taken in the authors' classes and has, over time, grown into the book you see here. The authors view the book as a tool for both undergraduate and graduate students, and it can be used as a stand-alone text or in combination with other materials. We hope you find the examples and exercises helpful.

Purpose of the Book

This book has been developed with applied learning in mind. Faculty members can use the concepts and examples included in each chapter to teach students about strategic analysis, and then students can use the blank templates available in most of the chapters to apply the knowledge. Students are encouraged to choose a "project organization" at the outset and use the same organization for the sequence of in-depth exercises that runs from Chapter 5 to Chapter 25. We feel that, through the application of the material, students will gain a greater understanding of strategic analysis and strategic management and thus be better prepared to meet the demands of their future careers. We hope you find our approach both appealing and useful, and we thank you for using the book.

Michael S. Wayland
Methodist University
Fayetteville, North Carolina

Warren G. McDonald
Methodist University
Fayetteville, North Carolina

PART

I

APPROACHING STRATEGIC ANALYSIS

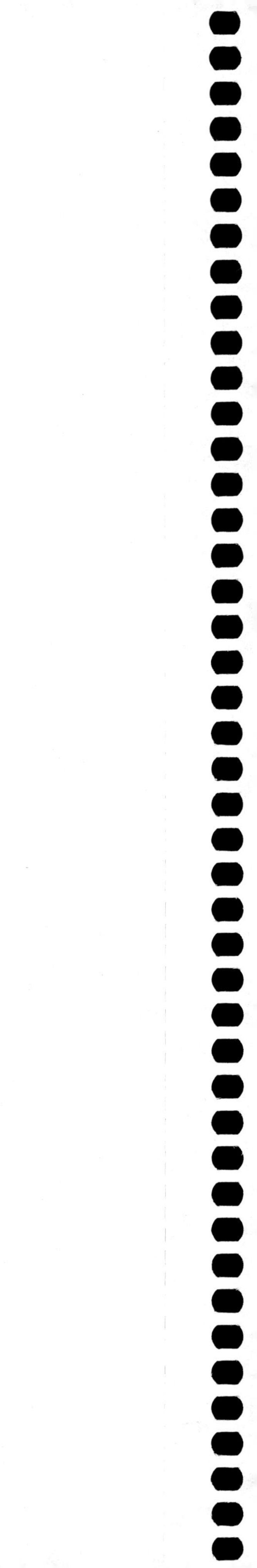

CHAPTER

1

INTRODUCTION TO BUSINESS STRATEGY

During the course of this book, you will encounter a variety of methods, matrices, and frameworks for strategic analysis, and you will gain firsthand experience in applying these tools in a series of exercises that builds from one chapter to the next. But before we delve into the sections on broad analysis, focused analysis, integrated analysis, strategy development, and strategy selection, we first need to understand the basics of business strategy.

The development of business strategy begins by asking three important questions:

1. Where are we now? (internal and external analysis)
2. Where do we want to be? (mission and strategy development)
3. How do we get there? (strategy development and implementation)

We begin the book by looking at questions 1 and 2: Where are we, and where do we want to be in the future? Answering these questions involves understanding the company's mission as it exists and reassessing it for where the company sees itself in the future. Understanding the company's current mission statement is sometimes straightforward but other times extremely difficult. Sometimes a mission statement is simply a plaque on the wall. Where the company really sees itself might be something completely different. We can think of no place that demands a higher degree of effective strategic management than healthcare, and we hope this book will help practitioners and students alike accomplish their goals more effectively.

Getting from today to a desired future state—the focus of question 3—is a difficult journey, and it depends on numerous factors, including how the organization sees itself, its competitors, its market, and so on. Goodstein, Nolan, and Pfeiffer (1993, 3) define applied strategic planning as "the process by which the guiding members of an organization envision its future and develop the necessary procedures and operations to achieve that future." Frequently, this process is neither easy nor well done. A *McKinsey Quarterly* survey of 2,207 executives revealed the following (Lovallo and Sibony 2010):

- 28 percent of executives surveyed said that the quality of strategic decisions in their companies was generally good.
- 60 percent thought that bad decisions were about as frequent as good ones.
- 12 percent thought good decisions were generally absent.

This book aims to help you in the challenging task of developing effective business strategy. The chapters are structured to guide you through understanding the company's mission statement, analyzing the external environment in which the firm competes, ana-

EXHIBIT 1.1 Business Strategy Development

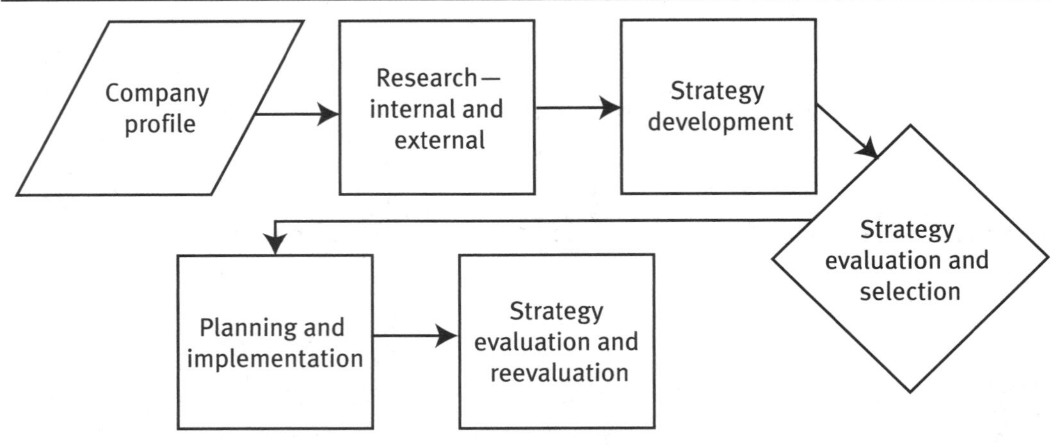

lyzing the internal environment of the company, and looking at the intersection of the inside and the outside. Once you have mastered these concepts, you will use the knowledge gained to create potential strategies, select the appropriate strategies, implement the desired strategies, and reevaluate the mission statement in light of the changes. The overall approach is illustrated in Exhibit 1.1.

References

Goodstein, L. D., T. M. Nolan, and J. W. Pfeiffer. 1993. *Applied Strategic Planning: How to Develop a Plan That Really Works.* New York: McGraw-Hill.

Lovallo, D., and O. Sibony. 2010. "The Case for Behavioral Strategy." *McKinsey Quarterly.* Published March. www.mckinsey.com/insights/strategy/the_case_for_behavioral_strategy.

CHAPTER

TEAM TECHNIQUES FOR STRATEGY DEVELOPMENT: BRAINSTORMING, FUTURE-PERFECT THINKING, AND AFFINITY CHARTS

2

Nolan, Goodstein, and Goodstein (2008, 2–3) write: "It is important to note that beginning a plan with a vision of a desired future for an organization leads to a very different outcome than that obtained from . . . an extrapolation of current business trends. Beginning with the present and planning a future very much like the present is a far cry from envisioning a desired future and planning how such a future can be achieved. Envisioning involves the conviction that our present actions can influence our future—we can help create our own future rather than passively accept whatever comes to pass. A powerful well-thought-out vision can become a magnet pulling an organization toward its ideal future."

The development of business strategy is rarely done alone; instead, it most often involves a strategy development team. This team is typically a cross-functional group that draws its members from such diverse areas of the company as human resources, finance, manufacturing, and sales. Thus, we should begin our study of the strategic planning process with a review of team techniques such as brainstorming, future-perfect thinking, and affinity charts.

Brainstorming

Brainstorming is a process for generating ideas in a group. The underlying concept is similar to the old adage that "two heads are better than one." If everyone involved (stakeholders) in a project, an issue, or a problem can come together and generate possible solutions, the variety of ideas will be greater, and the opportunity for a superior outcome is increased. Further, stakeholders are more likely to accept an outcome if they themselves had a hand in creating it. Brainstorming is particularly useful when creative, outside-the-box, or nonapparent solutions are needed.

Often, corporate or national cultures create barriers that prevent people from sharing their ideas openly and freely. For example, in an autocratic culture where people only do what they are told to, employees are less likely to speak up to voice opinions or make suggestions. In a highly critical culture, or in a culture that does not tolerate failure, people may be afraid to suggest a different way of doing things for fear of criticism. Brainstorming overcomes these barriers by creating an environment where it is not only safe but also expected for people to contribute their ideas.

The concept of brainstorming was introduced by advertising executive Alex F. Osborn in his 1963 book, *Applied Imagination: Principles and Procedures of Creative Problem Solving*. His four main principles of brainstorming were (1) to focus on quantity instead of quality, (2) to not allow criticism, (3) to welcome off-the-wall ideas, and (4) to encourage the group to improve ideas by building off the ideas of others. These core ideas still apply today.

To create a safe environment for idea generation, the brainstorming group usually begins by setting its own ground rules. The ground rules set the parameters and establish what the group finds to be acceptable and unacceptable. Typical ground rules may include the following:

1. No ideas are bad ideas; give any and all ideas you think of.
2. Speak one person at a time; don't speak over others.
3. Criticism of other people's ideas is not permitted.
4. Everyone participates.
5. Ideas will be evaluated only at the end, not as ideas are generated.
6. Think outside the box.

The purpose of brainstorming is to generate as many ideas as possible. Quality is not important; quantity is. The ground rules are usually developed with the aim of ensuring the maximum number of ideas. If a group member suggests an idea and the other group members immediately dissect it, evaluate it, and tear it apart, the person who put forward the idea may feel criticized and avoid offering similar ideas in the future. Furthermore, the group's time has now been refocused on determining how "meritorious" an idea was instead of on creating more ideas. The idea generation process has thus been inhibited.

Brainstorming can be formal or informal. One person is designated the "scribe," "facilitator," or "leader." This person has the role of writing down every idea generated. Usually the ideas are written on a flip chart. Alternatively, "sticky notes" or even a chalkboard can be used. Often, the scribe role rotates so that no one person dominates the process. Many groups will establish the principle that the scribe does not offer ideas but only writes. This rule is intended to prevent the scribe from exerting leadership that could direct or redirect the group's efforts toward a particular path.

Brainstorming begins with group members offering quick, brief ideas. Deep descriptions are not necessary. A brainstorm idea might sound like "What if we did X?" As an example, imagine an executive team that is trying to cut costs for the company. The first idea offered might be, "We could cut our workforce by 10 percent." Instead of judging the idea, the scribe jots it down and moves on to the next idea.

If the "cut our workforce" suggestion is attacked by a team member, the scribe reminds the group to hold off on evaluations and presses the group for more ideas. Even ridiculous and off-the-wall ideas are desired. Sometimes these "crazy" ideas have no value, but other times they can spur another person's mind to think of something new. Building off of other people's ideas is not considered cheating but rather a great way to generate additional ideas.

In our cost-cutting example above, the workforce reduction idea might lead to a suggestion to open the company's union contract for early renegotiation, which in turn might spur someone to think of renegotiating contracts with suppliers. This idea, in turn, might cause someone to suggest renegotiating contracts with customers. Someone else might suggest asking the leasing company that owns the headquarters office building to reduce the rent. Finally, someone might remember reading that the government had recently designated the inner-city area nearby as an enterprise zone, which would allow for tax incentives and state subsidies if the company moved its headquarters there. The idea generation process just moved from laying off employees to relocating the company headquarters!

With formal brainstorming, the group sits around a conference table. The participants offer ideas in the order in which they are sitting. Clarifying questions may be asked, but no commentary or evaluation is given. If a person has an idea, she must wait her turn to offer it. Team members are encouraged to write their ideas down on paper so they don't forget them. If an individual cannot think of an idea, he says "I pass," and his turn is skipped until it next comes around. Formal brainstorming has become rather uncommon, however.

Informal brainstorming has largely replaced formal brainstorming. Informal brainstorming allows all the essential components to remain in place, but the group members do not offer ideas in a specified order. Anyone can shout out an idea at any time. This process may be more chaotic, but it often yields more ideas. It also requires a scribe or leader who can successfully manage the group dynamics and keep the group from derailing.

Brainstorming is expected to generate a significant number of ideas. The sheer volume of ideas suggests that not all ideas will be viable. In later chapters, we will discuss analytical and quantitative methods of evaluating alternate strategies. For now, we can look at some simple approaches for retaining and discarding brainstormed ideas.

Following the idea generation session, the team members will work to reduce the number of ideas to a manageable group. Initially, the group will likely agree that certain ideas are clearly not viable, even without discussing the value of the ideas. These can be immediately discarded. Some ideas will have mixed support. These ideas will likely lead to a debate over their merits. Finally, some ideas may have immediate unanimous appeal.

Often, brainstorming facilitators will bring small, sticky circle labels and distribute three to each team member. The team members then place the sticky labels next to the three ideas they most strongly support. The ideas that attract the most votes will remain; the other ideas will be held in reserve as backups or will simply be discarded.

Future-Perfect Thinking

Future-perfect thinking finds its origins in phenomenological philosophy and how we know the nature of reality. Lindaman and Lippitt (1979) found that when people planned backward from the future to the present, they developed more robust, exciting, and committed plans. Future-perfect thinking is a planning tool in which group members pick a particular date at some point in the future, imagine they are actually there, imagine the perfect scenario, and then work backward from that point in order to determine how they "actually" got there. For example, imagine you are five years in the future and your company has 70 percent market share, up from 37 percent. How did the company do it? What was done to get there?

In essence, future-perfect thinking involves projecting oneself into a perfect future situation and then imagining how it occurred. The theory behind future-perfect thinking is that when you project yourself into the future, all the things that occurred between now and that future are part of the "past." Psychological studies have shown that people tend to be able to describe the events of the past more fully and accurately than they can describe future possibilities. By projecting yourself into the future, actu-

EXHIBIT 2.1
Affinity Chart, Step 1: Develop Multiple Ideas

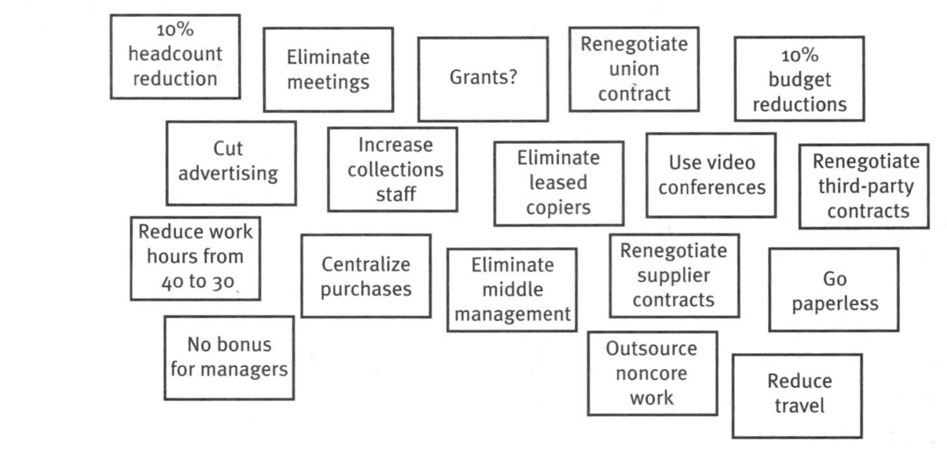

ally imagining yourself there, and describing it as perfect, you can more effectively identify the "past" events that led to it. You can more clearly describe the steps toward that perfect future than if you simply envisioned where you are today and decided what strategies to employ next.

The process of determining "what happened" can be a discussion or a debate, or it can incorporate principles of brainstorming. All the ideas are recorded, and the path to the perfect future situation is mapped out. Plans are then enacted to achieve the desired outcome.

Affinity Charts

An affinity chart is a method of organizing the data generated in brainstorming. An affinity chart takes the aggregate data generated and looks for similarities in the ideas. Ideas are grouped by similarity. A header is developed for each common group, and the ideas of that group are listed under the heading. Exhibits 2.1 to 2.4 demonstrate the steps in using affinity charts.

Step 1 in the process is to develop multiple ideas. In the example of cutting costs presented earlier, the ideas generated through brainstorming might be represented in the collection of sticky notes shown in Exhibit 2.1.

Step 2 is to group the ideas by some common concept. This step is illustrated in Exhibit 2.2.

Step 3 is to develop headings, as shown in Exhibit 2.3.

Step 4, represented in Exhibit 2.4, is to formalize.

Often in strategy development, the heading becomes the overarching strategy, and the ideas beneath the heading become the supporting strategies or even tactics to achieve the supporting strategies. In our example, an overarching strategy could be "Utilize operations actions to cut costs." Supporting strategies could include reducing layers of middle management, centralizing purchasing, outsourcing noncore work to suppliers, and increasing staff to reduce days in collection.

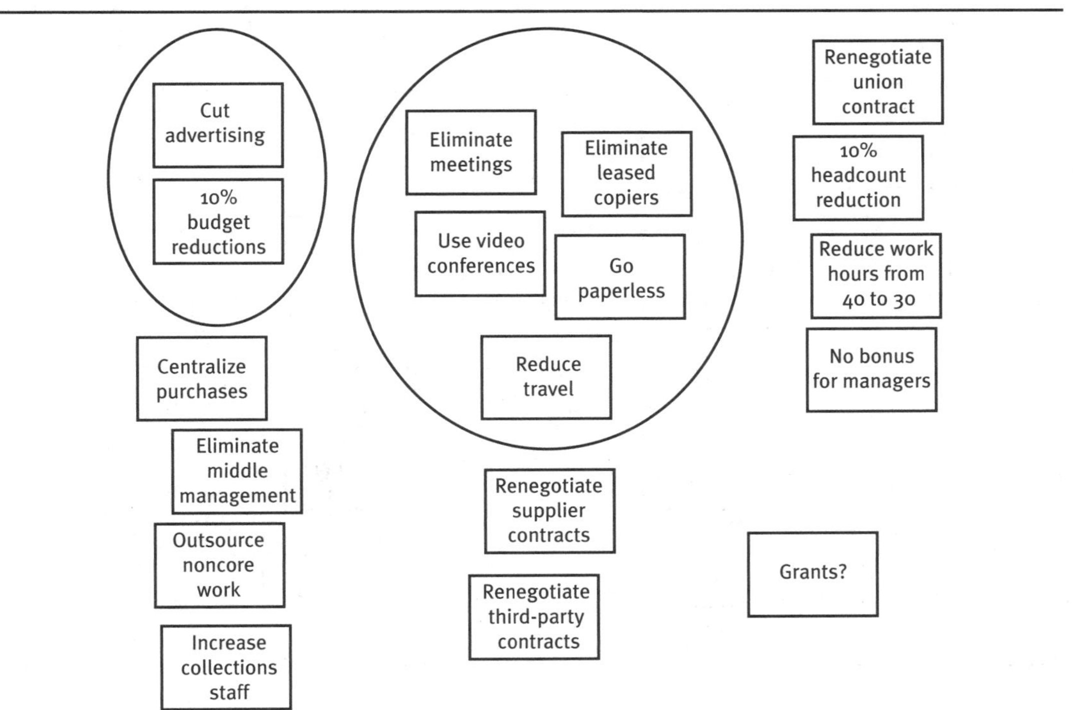

EXHIBIT 2.2
Affinity Chart, Step 2: Group by Common Concept

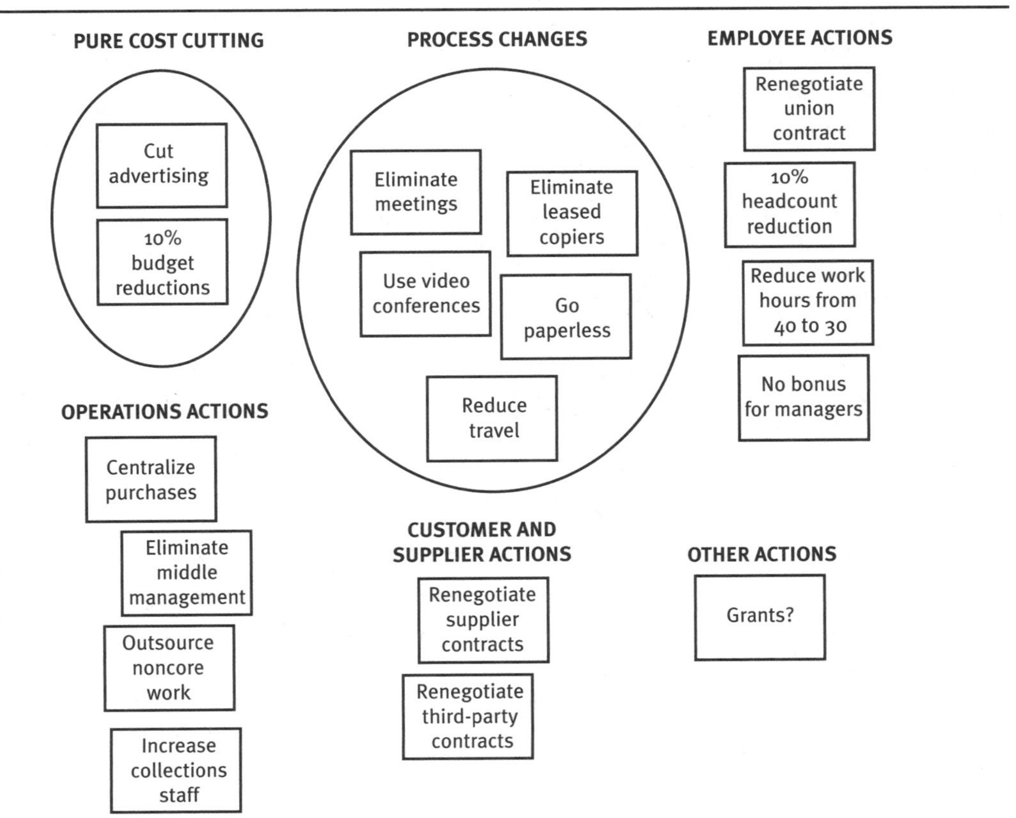

EXHIBIT 2.3
Affinity Chart, Step 3: Develop Headings

EXHIBIT 2.4
Affinity Chart, Step 4: Formalize

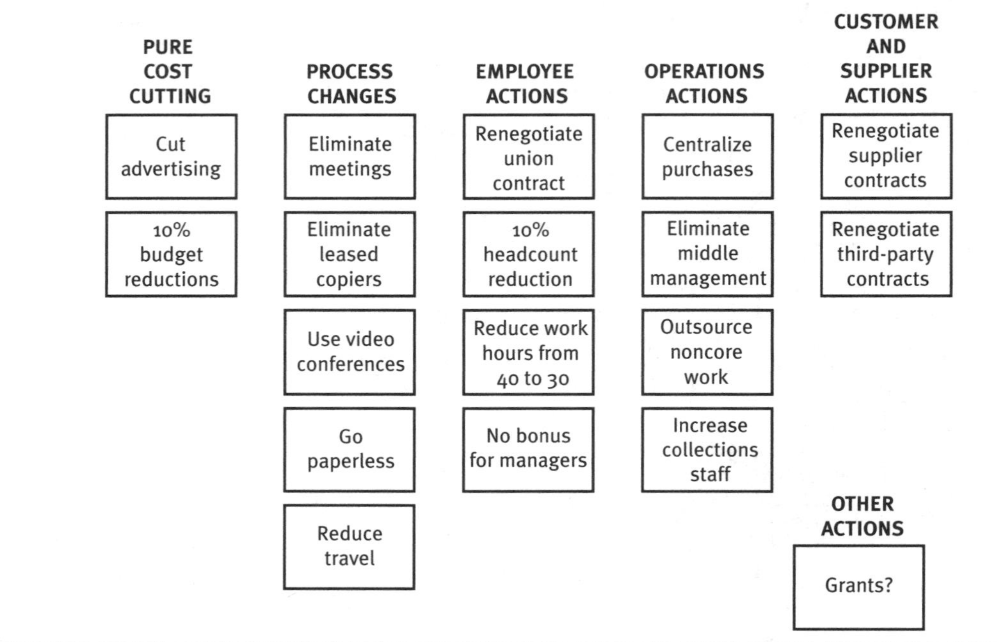

References

Lindaman, E. B., and R. O. Lippitt. 1979. *Choosing the Future You Prefer*. Washington, DC: Development Publications.

Nolan, T. M., L. D. Goodstein, and J. Goodstein. 2008. *Applied Strategic Planning: An Introduction*, 2nd ed. Hoboken, NJ: Wiley.

Osborn, A. F. 1963. *Applied Imagination: Principles and Procedures of Creative Problem Solving*. New York: Charles Scribner's Sons.

CHAPTER

3

RESEARCH AND COMPETITIVE ANALYSIS

Research and competitive analysis efforts allow you to find, collect, and understand a wide variety of important information about your business environment and your competitors. The Strategic and Competitive Intelligence Professionals association explains that there are five stages in what it calls the "intelligence cycle" (Weiss 2002):

1. Planning and direction
2. Published information collection
3. Primary source collection (personal interviews)
4. Analysis and production
5. Reporting and informing

Additionally, there are four potential types of competitors (Weiss 2002):

1. Organizations offering the same or similar products and services now
2. Organizations offering alternative products and services now
3. Organizations that could offer the same, similar, or alternative products and services in the future
4. Organizations that could remove the need for a product or service

Strategic analysts need to monitor other companies and study the overall business environment in which the company and its competitors operate. The ability to adapt to a changing environment before competitors do can be the key to a significant competitive advantage.

In this chapter, John McGonagle, managing partner of The Helicon Group, offers an overview of corporate and competitive analysis.

How to Approach Corporate and Competitive Analysis

by John McGonagle

In the past, competitive analysis—or, as it is more commonly called, competitive intelligence analysis—has largely been the responsibility of specialists within businesses, as is also the case in government. However, that arrangement is changing for a variety of reasons that are beyond the scope of this chapter. Nevertheless, you should look at corporate and competitive analysis, competitive intelligence, and similar disciplines as sources of additional tools for you to use individually.

There are five basic issues involved in conducting your own competitive analysis. First, what are you looking for, and why? Second, what limits are there on your research? Third, where might the necessary information—which in the field of competitive intelligence is called *data*—be located? Fourth, having at least initially determined where that data may be located, how do you get it? Fifth, once you have it, how do you make sense of the data so you can use it?

What Are You Looking for, and Why?

Answering this question is actually more difficult than it seems. Many researchers try to collect everything that exists out there, which is an endless and ultimately pointless task. Instead, you have to step back and define your new research. What specific intelligence are you looking for? A better way to phrase the question is this: If you had the intelligence that you are looking for, what decision would you be able to make that you cannot make without the intelligence? In other words, what is actionable? If you cannot answer this question, then your task is not refined enough. You risk seeking and then getting general information rather than actionable intelligence.

In addition, you should ask yourself, "Why do I want this intelligence? Is it to better understand the competitor?" If so, and if you wish to proceed on that basis, the amount of effort dedicated to that intelligence should be fairly small. If the purpose is to help conduct a more complex "war game," the research has to be more in depth and also must include more original material—such as advertisements, biographies, and interviews—rather than mere summaries of secondary materials. If you are trying to figure out your competitors' intentions and capabilities, you will have to look not only at brick and mortar but at people as well. People make decisions; buildings and invested capital do not.

Before going further, you should look around, literally and figuratively. Ask yourself, "Do I already have some of this data? If I do, should I use it? Is the data both reliable and current?" If so, you have at least a starting point. If the data is not current, it still might provide you with an indication of where you might seek the data today, as well as potential people to contact. If the data is not reliable, treat it as such.

What Are the Limits on Your Research?

Limits on your research can be many and varied. In evaluating them, you have to be coldly critical. Constraints to consider include the following:

- Just how much time can you devote to this research? The time is a function not only of your schedule but also of the importance of the intelligence that you could produce.
- What kind of resources do you have available? In other words, how much money can you spend; how much help can you get from others within your organization; and do you have an outside research company you can turn to for assistance?
- How might the calendar limit your research? Your deadline may be an important constraint. Remember, a pretty good answer that arrives on time might be better than a perfect one two weeks later.

A number of other constraints are less tangible. Such constraints are found within your own company's written and unwritten policies, as well as within legal and ethical considerations.

You should always check your company's policies on data collection. Some companies, for reasons unrelated to competitive intelligence, may prohibit you from actually calling a competitor. Such policies are likely due to historical concerns about antitrust issues. Some companies may have narrower prohibitions, such as telling their employees that they may not discuss pricing issues with any competitor. This type of rule is obviously to avoid price fixing. Whatever the limits are, you owe it to yourself and your employer to be aware of them and to abide by them.

The legal and ethical limits on competitive intelligence deal mainly with how information is collected. One should not steal materials from a competitor, misrepresent for whom one works, pretend to be a student doing a paper, or take any of a number of other dubious, even if not technically illegal, steps. Note that most of these issues actually fall within the realm of ethics, not the law.

The only legal regime directly applicable to competitive intelligence is the Economic Espionage Act of 1996. This act deals with the theft of trade secrets. If you come into possession of a trade secret of a competitor, the safest thing to do is to immediately contact your employer's attorneys, bring them all the materials that you may have received accidentally or otherwise, and let them handle the situation.

Most companies that have a competitive intelligence unit have a set of standards governing the unit's performance. If your company has such a unit, even if you are doing the work on your own, you are bound by whatever the unit's rules are. For an idea of the range of issues that surround the ethical collection of competitive intelligence, you may want to look at the Code of Ethics issued by the Strategic and Competitive Intelligence Professionals at www.scip.org.

Where Might the Data Be Located?

Before starting the search for the data you seek, first sit back for a moment and consider where the data may be located. Data, or information, is a "sticky" commodity. In other words, someone who has been in possession of some piece of data at one time still has a part of it even when it is passed on. That part of the data may be in the form of a copy of a document or in the individual's own memory.

One way to start your research is to determine where similar data about your own company is located. Having found where your company's data exists in the public domain, or at least where it is accessible to diligent research, you are better prepared to find similar data on your competitors.

You should first determine the most likely place that the *exact* data you need could be. Do not be limited by considerations of whether you have the ability to access that location. Rather, you are trying to understand where the data originates so that you can then determine, or at least estimate, how it moves from the original source to other places. These other locations may be within the competitor or outside the company. They may be employees, consultants, customers, suppliers, catalogs, surveys, and so on.

Your goal is to understand how the data moves and find out who changes, consolidates, or divides that data; then determine if and how you can approach these sources. You may find that the data you seek is not available from any one source but has been divided up among several. Such a situation is typical of pricing information. In these cases, you will have to approach several sources and (re)aggregate the data you collect. Only after you have made an effort to understand the origins and flow of data should you begin to seek it.

Listing resources and potential resources allows you to control your research. I am often asked how to tell when one has run out of places to look for data. My answer is to keep an inventory of the places and people approached or identified as sources for the data, even if you have not approached them yet. When you find that, as your research continues, new sources are referring you back to your old sources, you can usually assume that your research is done.

How Do You Get the Data?

Getting the data, as we have stated, requires having at least some idea of where the data might be located. Generally, you should start collecting secondary data before moving on to primary data (i.e., interviews and the like). The secondary data will provide you with a historical look at the subject or target. The secondary data should be reviewed for the names of individuals and organizations that you, or someone working for you outside your firm, may wish to contact for further information. This review can often lead to experts quoted in an article, an executive of a competitor who is no longer there, a supplier, or even a regulator.

The Internet should be viewed as a tool for obtaining data, but not as the source for all your data. You can usually get information faster from secondary sources on the Internet than you can otherwise. Business and social networking groups can help you identify and contact potential interviewees. For example, if you are trying to identify someone who is an intern at a particular company, a Facebook or LinkedIn page might be useful. Business networking pages can help you identify not only individuals for possible contact but, more importantly, individuals who formerly worked with the target. A former employee may not always have current information, but she almost always has information that is more valuable than that found in dated print sources.

Do not forget to look within your own organization. Ask if there are people who formerly worked at a competitor who now work for you. When approaching them, be clear that they are not obligated to talk about their work at their former employer, and that no one is putting pressure on them. What you want is full cooperation. If they feel constrained for ethical or even legal reasons, end the conversation. A key goal in any interview or attempted interview, whether internal or external, is to get another name that you can contact, preferably using the name of the person you spoke to as a reference. Opening the door in that manner is extremely valuable to developing useful primary information.

How Do You Make Sense of the Data So You Can Use It?

Once you (a) have run out of time, (b) have run out of budget, or (c) are being referred back to previous sources by individuals you interview or try to interview, you have "closed the loop." This point usually marks the end of well-conducted research, whether or not you have all the data you need.

Now, you must break the mind-set that has arisen during the data collection. You have collected data in a certain order, which is almost certainly neither chronological nor topical. The individuals you have interviewed were available on their schedule, not in an order chosen by you. So try the techniques below before determining what it is you actually think you have found.

First, order your information and notes chronologically—that is, in order of the time they reference. Now go back and read them, both from the oldest to newest and the newest to oldest. What gaps do you see? If you have time, consider conducting supplemental research to address the gaps.

Now, arrange your materials by topic, such as sales and marketing, production capabilities, personalities, and so on. Once again, look for gaps in your information. Again, see if supplemental research would be possible or valuable.

Now, put aside your research materials. Start writing what you think you know about the target, based on what you knew before you started your research (if you have time, do this writing at the start of the process). Put down your initial thoughts even if you believe your preconceptions have been contradicted or undercut by what you've learned.

Next, write out (or just outline, whichever you prefer) what you have learned from your research. Clearly identify things that are certain—confirmed facts—and distinguish them from your conclusions or inferences. We are not suggesting that your conclusions and inferences are not important; they are. But you should make a point to separate what you knew from what you know and from what you think you know.

Try to stand back from your research and look at it through someone else's eyes. If you don't have someone else working with you, the best you can do is to try to break through your own preconceptions, adopt a perspective different from your normal perspective, or use some other method to force yourself to stand back and think openly.

A wide variety of analytical tools are available once you have organized your data and reached your conclusions. However, you should select them only *after* you take a look at your data and conclusions. Do not start assuming you will be putting together a Boston Consulting Group matrix or a SWOT chart. Do not try to fit your facts and conclusions into one particular analytical model; rather, find a model that helps you deal best with the facts you have. Remember the old aphorism: "To a man with a hammer, everything looks like a nail."

In our case, because you are the end user of the research, a willingness to step back to break preconceptions, to change perspective, to be open to new views, and to challenge what you think you know becomes even more important than it would be in a normal competitive intelligence situation. There, a competitive intelligence specialist would report to an end user, which automatically provides for at least two perspectives on the research. When you are combining the roles of researcher, analyst, and customer into one, you must take extra care to avoid jumping to conclusions or blinding yourself to important anomalies to which you should pay attention.

Reference

Weiss, A. 2002. "A Brief Guide to Competitive Intelligence." *Business Information Review* 19 (2): 39–47.

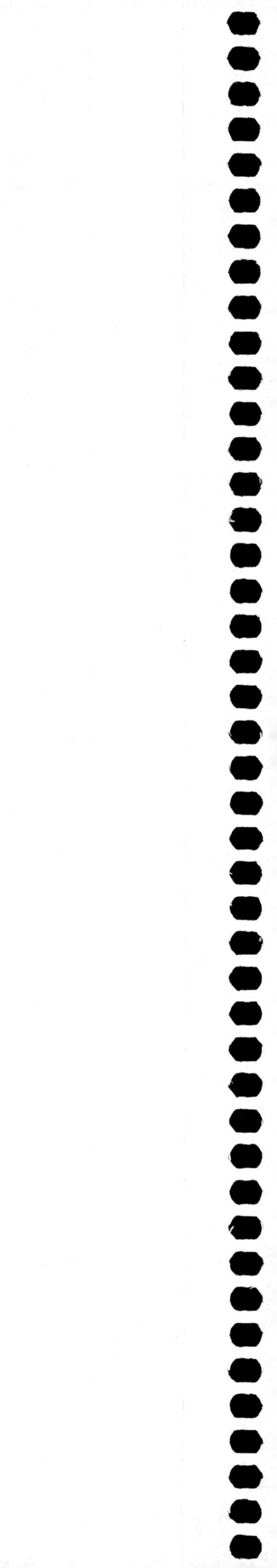

CHAPTER

4

CORPORATE MISSION

Your organization's mission is an essential part of strategy development. Notice we used the word *mission* as opposed to *mission statement*. The mission statement is just the verbal embodiment of the mission.

During the 1990s, organizational leaders would often spend days at an off-site meeting developing a mission statement. When they returned, they would share the statement with employees, hang a framed copy on the wall in the lobby, and then go on with life as usual. This approach had little impact on strategy or on the alignment of employee performance.

Contrast the above approach with that taken by the Frito-Lay company in the 1990s. Frito-Lay established a mission and mission statement of having salty snacks within an arm's reach of consumers anywhere in the world. It set four values, or "imperatives," by which it intended to reach that goal: *Cost*, *Quality*, *Service*, and *People*. *Cost* referred to all aspects of cost, from low manufacturing cost to reasonable retail cost. *Quality* referred to the highest quality in the industry, *Service* referred to the best possible customer service, and *People* represented treating employees well. These values became ingrained into the culture. You would be able to pull an hourly manufacturing employee off the production line and she could tell you the mission and values. In fact, she could tell you how she herself had an impact on cost, quality, service, and people!

Specific to healthcare, hospitals and other organizations also seek to contain significant cost increases, improve overall quality of healthcare and its delivery, and maximize human resources, which account for our most significant cost.

How Mission Affects Strategy

An organization's mission (e.g., salty snacks within an arm's reach of all consumers) leads directly to the conceptualization and development of strategy to achieve that mission. If the "salty snacks" example were your mission, what strategies could you think of to achieve it?

This "mission leads to strategy" linear thought process has limitations, however. The risk is that "the way we view the company now remains the way through which we develop strategy," and thus we miss the brand new ideas and new markets. Why couldn't Frito-Lay's mission statement have been to have salty snacks *and chocolate* within an arm's length of consumers? If the company's executives view the world of strategic possibilities solely through the lens of salty snacks, they might miss significant opportunities. This concern brings us to the proposition that the relationship between strategy and mission is

EXHIBIT 4.1
Circular Relationship Between Mission and Strategy

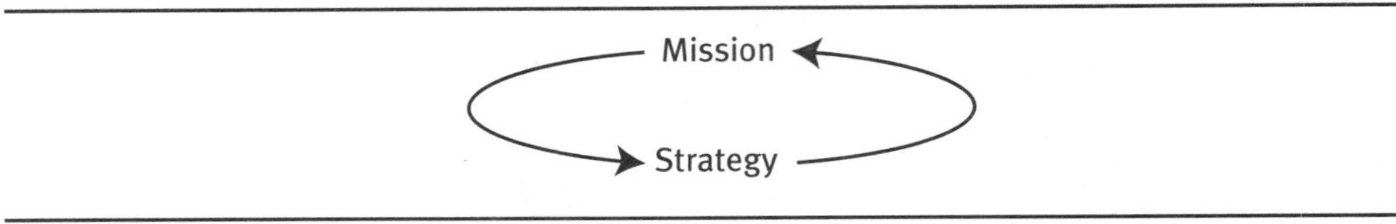

circular rather than linear—that is, though mission may lead to strategy, strategic analysis may lead to a revision of the mission and new strategic development (see Exhibit 4.1).

How to Develop a Corporate Mission

There are three distinct components to a well-constructed corporate mission. The first is the "pure" mission statement, second is the overarching vision, and third are the guiding principles:

- Our mission: what we do
- Our vision: where we are going
- Our values: how we will get there

Our Mission

This component describes what the company now does or is aspiring to do as a "go-forward" mission. It is shaped, limited, or stretched by how executives see or do not see themselves, the company, competitors, the industry, customers, and the economy. Ibarreche (2012) suggests considering the following issues: needs or wants; to whom, where, how; difference from competition; other sources of uniqueness; self-concept; external image; philosophy; people; other stakeholders; and quality.

Exhibit 4.2 provides an example of a mission statement from Dimensions Healthcare System. One can read this simple statement and clearly understand what this system does: "provide comprehensive healthcare of the highest quality to residents, and others . . . while strengthening our relationships with universities, research and healthcare organizations." The shorter, the easier to comprehend, and the easier to recall a mission is, the more effective it will be. The mission should not be three unmemorable paragraphs. Those missions end up framed, hung on a wall, and irrelevant in the everyday work, behavior, and decision making of employees and managers.

Our Vision

This component describes where we are going with the organization in the future. It is the *stretch* of the mission statement. As with all parts of the mission, the vision may be limited

EXHIBIT 4.2
Dimensions Healthcare System's Mission Statement

Mission statement: Within Dimensions Healthcare System it is our mission to provide comprehensive healthcare of the highest quality to residents, and others who use our services, while strengthening our relationships with universities, research and healthcare organizations to ensure best-in-class patient care.

Source: Dimensions Healthcare System (2015).

by a variety of factors. Consider that in the mid-1970s the executives at Sears believed that the retail industry was maxed out and provided little opportunity. This view constrained management's vision of retail, and it caused the leadership to consider other possibilities for growth. It directly led to the development of a nonretail strategy of expansion into financial services, the creation of the Discover credit card, the acquisition of the Dean Witter stock brokerage firm, and so on. Contrast this view of the retail industry with the view held by Sam Walton and his executives around the same time. Wal-Mart's view was that retail held unlimited possibilities, so its corporate vision was to maximize that existing opportunity. Wal-Mart's vision translated into an aggressive expansion strategy, and now the company is becoming a major player in healthcare as well.

In addition to describing where the organization is going in the future, the vision can get employees and investors excited, "bought in," and passionate about the chosen direction. Griswell and Jennings (2009) write that great business leaders compose corporate visions that are also intended to develop and engage passion in their employees. The leaders who get their corporate vision statements right are the ones who know how to align purpose and passion.

Griswell and Jennings point to Wal-Mart's mission: "To give ordinary folk the chance to buy the same thing as rich people." This vision of *empowering* the common person permeated the organization and excited the employees, causing them to believe they were doing something socially good, not just good for the organization. (Consider this vision in the context of the 1970s' hyperinflation and significantly greater income disparity between the "haves" and the "have nots.") The employees' passion to give people of limited financial means access to products and quality that previously were only accessible to people with greater wealth drove phenomenal growth from the 1970s to the 2010s. For evidence, just look at Wal-Mart's financial results. So many "ordinary folk" purchased products at Wal-Mart that it became one of the top businesses in the United States and has expanded internationally. Wal-Mart is now seeking to be a leading provider of primary care in America, with in-store clinics staffed by mid-level providers. In some regards, Wal-Mart has always been in healthcare via its deeply discounted pharmacies, but now it is expanding its approach.

Having the right vision is central to creating the employee passion that drives business results. Passion, in turn, can be thought of as the enthusiasm employees feel from being a part of the company's vision. Who does not want to be a part of changing the world or, from a business perspective, helping take a company from average to number one?

Dimensions Healthcare System's vision statement (see Exhibit 4.3) clearly articulates where the organization is going in the future: The organization wishes to be recognized as a premier regional provider. Beyond clearly stating an outlook for the future, this vision might also include opportunities to expand even further as development continues—for example, becoming the top-rated system in the country, and even global expansion.

EXHIBIT 4.3
Dimensions Healthcare System's Vision Statement

Vision: To be recognized as a premier regional health care system.

Source: Dimensions Healthcare System (2015).

EXHIBIT 4.4
Dimensions Healthcare System's Values

Dimensions Healthcare System:

- Respects the dignity and privacy of each patient who seeks our service.
- Is committed to excellent service which exceeds the expectations of those we serve.
- Accepts and demands personal accountability for the services we provide.
- Consistently strives to provide the highest quality work from individual performance.
- Promotes open communication to foster partnership and collaboration.
- Is committed to an innovative environment; encouraging new ideas and creativity.
- Is committed to having its hospitals meet the highest standards of safety.

Source: Dimensions Healthcare System (2015).

Our Values (Guiding Principles)

The third component describes how the organization will achieve the mission and vision. The values are guiding principles that inform employees and constrain actions (to the extent that management truly believes them and holds people accountable). Values may involve such areas as fiscal responsibility, respect for employees, quality, and environmental responsibility. Actions that violate the values will be rejected by employees, and actions that are consistent with the values will survive. Dimensions Healthcare System's values are shown in Exhibit 4.4.

An employee who understands the organization's values and sees them reinforced by management will clearly realize the commitment to high integrity and customer satisfaction. Conformance to the values will be significantly higher than if the values had not been articulated.

Bringing It All Together

Exhibit 4.5 shows an example of a corporate mission taken from EmergingLeader.com (2014). Though the organization is not in the healthcare field, its mission provides a clear and concise example we can use here as a guide.

EXHIBIT 4.5
Example of Corporate Mission

Our Mission:
To provide a forum for leadership improvement through user participation and submissions. No matter what stage you have reached in perfecting your leadership style, we have something for you.

Our Vision:
To continue to grow, improve and provide our customers with the best information for the betterment of their own leadership skills.

Guiding Principles:
We utilize Honor, Courage, Commitment and Integrity to guide our decisions and help us keep perspective.

Source: EmergingLeader.com (2014).

References

Dimensions Healthcare System. 2015. "Mission, Vision, Values." Accessed June 16. www.dimensionshealth.org/index.php/about-us/mission-vision-values/.

EmergingLeader.com. 2014. "Mission, Vision, and Guiding Principles." Accessed December 1. www.EmergingLeader.com/mvgp.htm.

Griswell, J. B., and B. Jennings. 2009. *The Adversity Paradox: An Unconventional Guide to Achieving Uncommon Business Success*. New York: St. Martin's Press.

Ibarreche, S. 2012. *Strategic Management: Using Ideas in Action*. Dubuque, IA: Kendall Hunt.

Consider the following information from the website of the Christiana Care Health System (2015). Read through it all, and then develop a mission statement for the organization in the space provided.

EXERCISE

About Christiana Care Health System

Christiana Care Health System, headquartered in Wilmington, Delaware, is one of the country's largest health care providers, ranking 22nd in the nation for hospital admissions.

Christiana Care is a major teaching hospital with two campuses and more than 250 Medical-Dental residents and fellows. Christiana Care is recognized as a regional center for excellence in cardiology, cancer and women's health services. The system is home to Delaware's only Level I trauma center, the only center of its kind between Philadelphia and Baltimore. Christiana Care also features a Level III neonatal intensive care unit, the only delivering hospital in the state to offer this level of care for newborns.

A not-for-profit, non-sectarian health system, Christiana Care includes two hospitals with more than 1,100 patient beds, a home health care service, preventive medicine, rehabilitation services, a network of primary care physicians and an extensive range of outpatient services.

With more than 10,500 employees, Christiana Care is the largest private employer in Delaware and the 10th largest employer in the Philadelphia region. In fiscal year 2013, Christiana Care had $2.51 billion in total patient revenue and provided the community with $26.8 million in charity care (at cost).

Statistics at a Glance

Among hospitals in the United States, Christiana Care's ranking by volume is:

- 21st in admissions.
- 29th in births.
- 24th in emergency visits.
- 24th in total surgeries.

Among hospitals on the East Coast, Christiana Care ranks:

- 11th in admissions.
- 13th in births.
- 12th in emergency visits.
- 12th in total surgeries.

(*Source*: American Hospital Association Annual Survey Database of 6,200 U.S. Hospitals, FY 2012, © Health Forum, LLC)

Fiscal Year 2013 Statistics for Christiana Care Health System

Admissions	52,779
Emergency Department Visits	181,237
Home Health Care Visits	307,172
Births	6,427

(continued)

EXERCISE

Surgical Procedures	38,803
Open Heart Cases	682
Radiology Procedures	389,568
Rehabilitation Patients	659
Rehabilitation Services Visits	106,178
Total Hip and Knee Replacements	2,536
Clinical Research Studies	886
Employees	10,834
Volunteers	1,202
Medical-Dental Staff	1,496
Medical-Dental Residents and Fellows	282

The Christiana Care Way

The Christiana Care Way is our promise to you—and to each other: "We serve our neighbors as respectful, expert, caring partners in their health. We do this by creating innovative, effective, affordable systems of care that our neighbors value."

As a not-for-profit health system, our mission is one of service. We believe that the key to providing truly great health care is to partner with our patients and their families, building a system of care that is effective, affordable and valuable to everyone who is touched by it.

How do we know what is valuable to our patients? We ask. And we listen. We understand that medical expertise is fully effective only when it is paired with respect and compassion. And we understand that the way to help our neighbors to get well and to stay that way requires that we take the time to learn about who they are, what they want, and what they need.

The Christiana Care Way is also an invitation to you. As a patient or a visitor, or as a member of our community, we welcome you as a partner. Tell us how we're doing, and let us know if you've had a good experience or if you see an opportunity for us to do something better.

We invite you to learn more about The Christiana Care Way. You can find out more about why each word was chosen. And you can see it in the smiles and dedication of our physicians, nurses and support staff, who exemplify The Christiana Care Way every day.

Reference

Christiana Care Health System. 2015. "About Christiana Care Health System." Accessed June 16. www.christianacare.org/whoweare.

EXERCISE

Christiana Care Health System

Our Mission: What We Do

Our Vision: Where We Are Going

Our Values: How We Will Get There

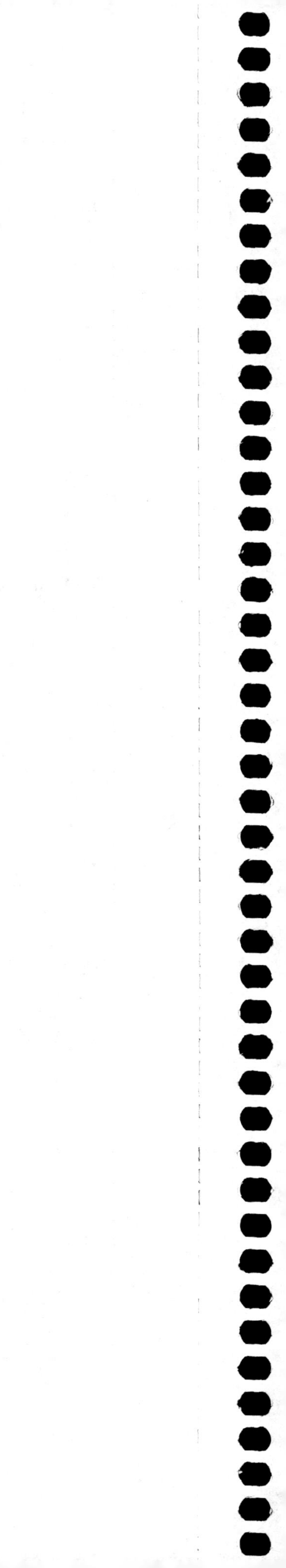

PART

BROAD ANALYSIS

CHAPTER

5

STRATEGIC INDUSTRY MAP

Before you can begin to analyze the strengths of your organization and develop corresponding strategy, you need to understand the industry in which you operate. To begin, many strategists will use a strategic industry map. The industry map allows you to view your industry by size and category.

The industry map attempts to capture a snapshot of an entire industry in a way that allows for one quick glance to provide a high level of information. First, a matrix is created. The matrix will have two axes with two variables. Typically, one axis will have some combination of price/quality/image, and the other axis will have some measure of product mix. The analyst chooses any labels felt to be appropriate.

Exhibit 5.1 shows the beginning of an industry map for healthcare in a local community, and its structure may mirror that of your own map.

Once the horizontal and vertical axes have been defined, the analyst identifies all the different industry segments. Using the clothing industry as an example, one might identify a number of segments ranging from custom-made-clothing tailors to mass-market retailers such as Wal-Mart. As we discussed in the previous chapter, Wal-Mart has expanded its reach with in-store clinics, so it now appears on the healthcare map as well. In healthcare, we look at everything from these new "doc-in-a-box" locations to private practices to hospital systems. We must include all segments of the industry to gain a clear perspective on our position in the marketplace.

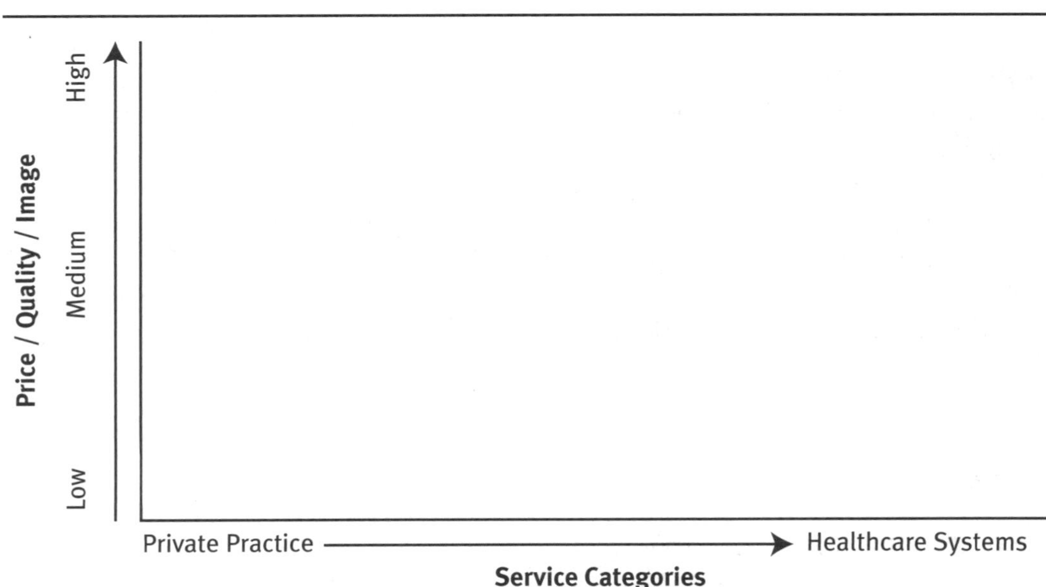

EXHIBIT 5.1
Beginning of a Strategic Industry Map

EXHIBIT 5.2 Strategic Map of the Healthcare Industry

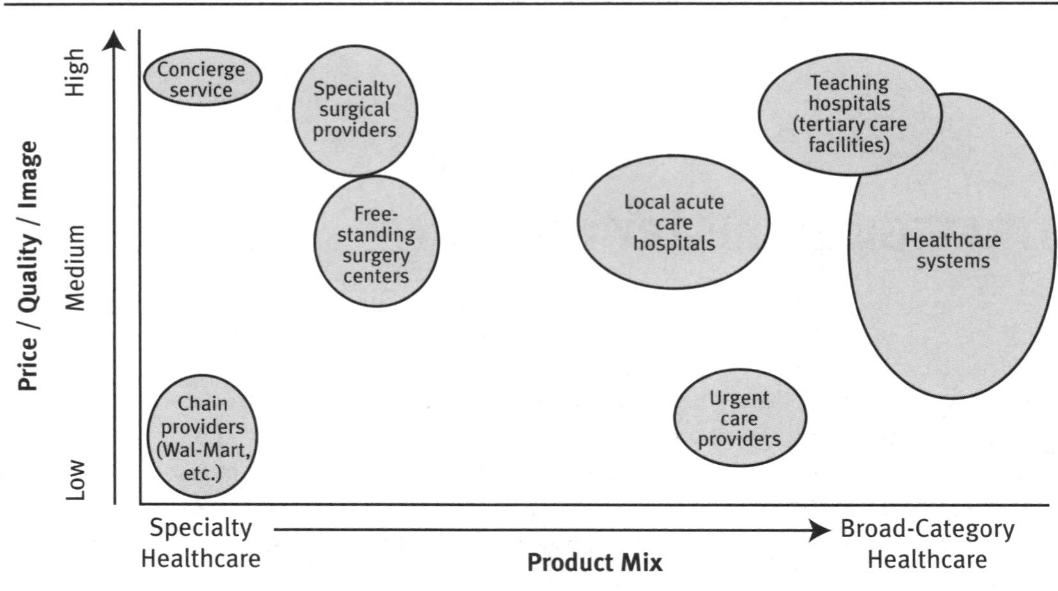

Each industry segment is represented by a circle on the matrix, and each circle is placed at the appropriate intersection of the two axes. The size of each circle represents the size of the industry segment relative to the other segments. Some analysts will include the projected dollar volume of each segment in parentheses immediately following the segment's name—for instance, "Mini-clinics ($250,000)," meaning that "mini-clinic" retail providers account for $250,000 in sales in the industry locally.

The example industry map in Exhibit 5.2 displays the different size, quality, image, and product attributes of major players in healthcare. Note that the circles represent industry segments, not specific organizations. Specific organizations can be included in parentheses simply to typify the segment.

Notice the area in the map that represents the intersection of low price and specialty care. Is there a business opportunity there for an entrepreneurial provider? At one time there was.

When that corner of the map was unfilled, stores such as Wal-Mart, CVS, and Walgreens saw a demand for primary care and developed local walk-in clinics at many of their locations. Time will tell how such efforts are received, but initial signs suggest they are successful.

Kim and Maugborgne (2005) identified wide-open gaps in the industry map as "blue oceans"—uncontested spaces where no one competes. "Red oceans" are places where competition already exists and has left "blood in the water." "Blue ocean strategy" involves seeking out uncontested market space and providing new market offerings. Under those circumstances, the lack of competition can lead to quicker market dominance and higher profits.

Reference

Kim, W. C., and R. Maugborgne. 2005. *Blue Ocean Strategy: How to Create Uncontested Market Space and Make the Competition Irrelevant.* Boston: Harvard Business Review Press.

EXERCISE

Create an industry map using the blank map provided. For this exercise and the exercises in later chapters, you will use a project organization of your choosing. Your project organization can be an organization with which you are currently associated or any other organization you wish to use in the book's exercises.

1. *Identify the industry your organization is a part of, and title your map appropriately.*
2. *Identify the appropriate axis labels to use on your map, such as price versus breadth of product mix.*
3. *Identify the market segments within the market. Note that you are identifying market segments, not brands.*
4. *Identify the size of each market segment.*
5. *Identify the attributes of each segment.*
6. *Place each market segment on the map, using the size of the circle to represent the size of the segment in dollar volume. Use the location on the map to correspond to the attributes you identified.*

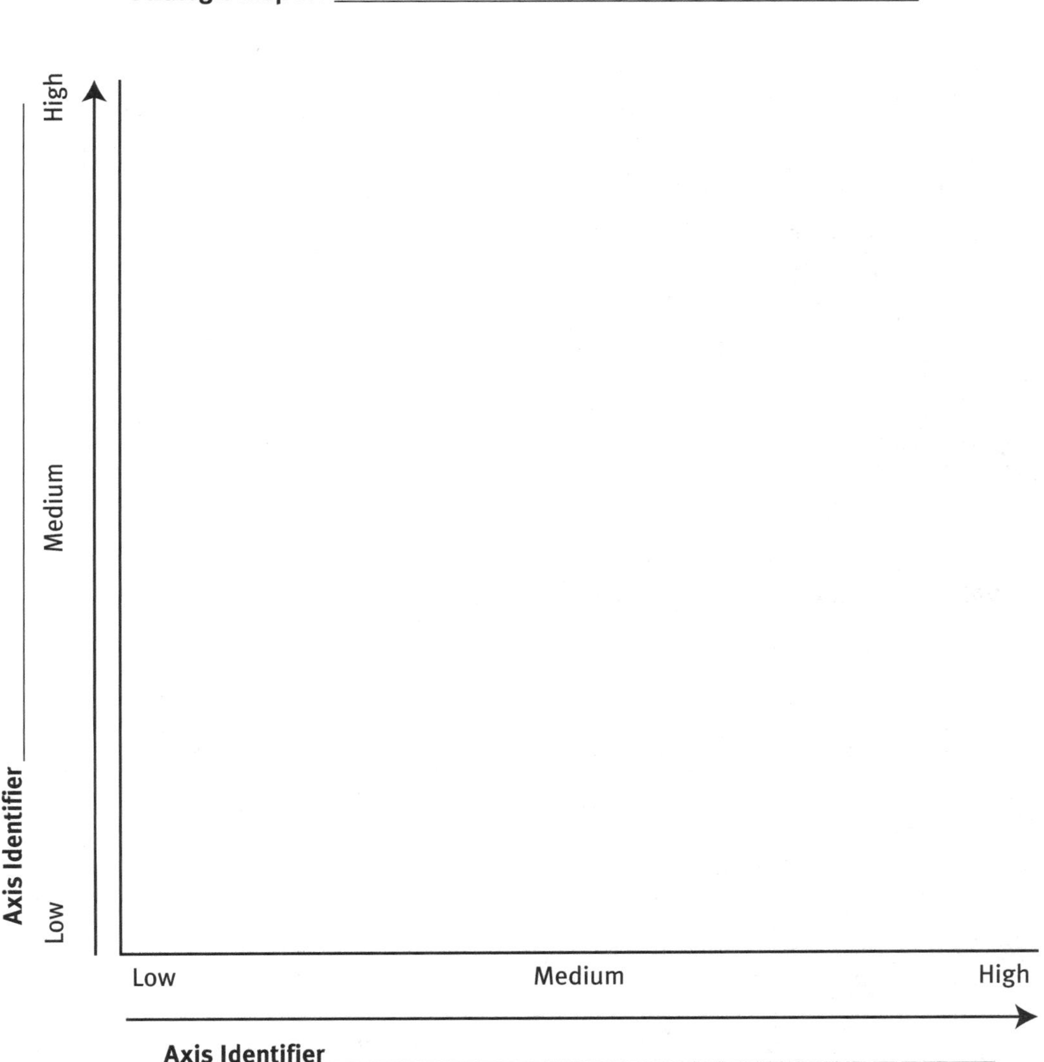

EXERCISE

After completing the map of your industry, answer the following questions:

1. Do you see any weaknesses in the industry?

2. How about opportunities?

3. Are there any "blue oceans"?

4. What implications for strategy development does the industry map provide?

CHAPTER

6

FIVE FORCES IN AN INDUSTRY

Five forces analysis is a popular approach to analyzing industry factors that are likely to affect strategy. It was developed by Michael Porter (1980) and made popular in his book *Competitive Strategy: Techniques for Analyzing Industries and Competitors*. While the approach is decades old, it remains significant, widely used, and highly applicable to healthcare. The five forces shape, constrain, and provide opportunities for competitive advantage for your organization. The forces influence how profitable a business in the particular industry will be, how much reasonable investment can be made into the industry, and how much growth opportunity exists in that industry. The five forces are (1) threat of entry, (2) intensity of rivalry, (3) threat of substitute products, (4) bargaining power of suppliers, and (5) bargaining power of buyers. The forces are shown in Exhibit 6.1 and discussed in detail in the sections that follow.

Threat of Entry

The threat of new competitors entering a given market is one industry force that affects strategy. If a company invests billions of dollars to create a new product that can be easily imitated by new entrants in the market, where is the competitive advantage? There may be some advantages—such as the profit made while a potential new entrant is still developing its product, goodwill among customers, or the building of a top-of-mind brand name—but as we will see in later chapters, a sustainable "first mover" advantage does not always exist. On the other hand, if competitors are hard-pressed to enter the market, a significant competitive advantage may exist for your company to move into the market first. If your

EXHIBIT 6.1
Five Forces

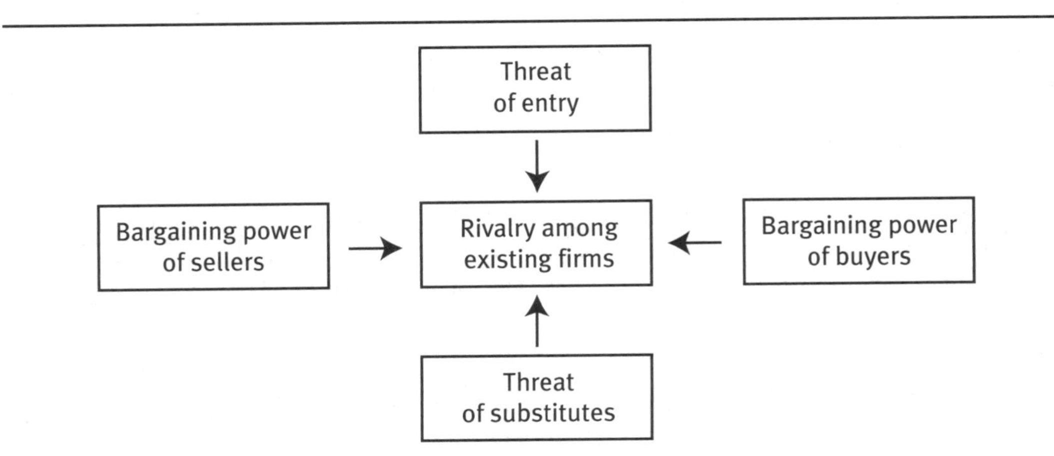

EXHIBIT 6.2
Potential Barriers to Market Entry

1. Capital requirements
2. Supplier industry manufacturing over capacity
3. Economies of scale
4. Government regulation, tax, tariffs, protectionism
5. Established brands
6. Switching costs
7. Access to distribution channels
8. Advertising, marketing, and promotion costs
9. Product interchangeability

company is in an existing market, analysis of the threat of entry can help you ascertain your ability to maintain your market share and prepare defensive strategies to prevent a potential new competitor from arising.

Threat of entry can be considered in terms of two main factors: (1) barriers to entry and (2) response of existing competitors. Exhibit 6.2 shows some potential barriers to entry. If there is one supplier of a critical component and your company has a contractually exclusive arrangement with that supplier, if a resource is scarce and you have it controlled, or if the dollar investment is prohibitively high for a competitor to justify entering the market, one would say the barrier to entry for a new entrant is high. In healthcare, cost is an especially significant barrier, as costs to establish a new healthcare product or service are typically high due to a variety of factors (regulations by the Food and Drug Administration, for instance). Conversely, if you are dealing with broadly and inexpensively available commodities, easy technology, and consumer indifference to brand, the barrier to entry for a new competitor is low. We have seen this effect in the eye care industry, with new online providers offering contact lenses and glasses at greatly reduced prices.

Competitor responsiveness can lower the threat of entry if the existing competitors are well funded, have the ability to leverage well-established brand names, can aggressively cut prices and maintain low profit margins that would put new competitors out of business, or have a willingness to "defend their turf." Organizations will be less likely to invest large sums of money in a venture that might not get off the ground or might fail to deliver a generous rate of return on investment.

Does this scenario exist in contemporary healthcare? Of course. We are seeing the systemization of healthcare organizations to ensure some level of dominance in the markets they serve. Individual hospitals have little chance of competing with the larger healthcare systems today, so they attempt to keep others out of their markets by becoming larger and stronger.

Intensity of Rivalry

Some have said that there is no such thing as a sustainable competitive advantage, because your competitors will always find a way to mimic or copy anything that succeeds for you. If you buy new technology for your operation, the suppliers, or their competitors, will tout their equipment to your competitors, citing your purchase. If you invent a new product, your competitors will at some point find a way around your patents with a similar product. The intensity of rivalry among existing industry competitors drives this imitation strategy. This intensity can be easily seen in many industries, including healthcare. The higher the intensity, the more difficult it will be for your company to profit and grow in the market. A high intensity will also dictate a strong need for defensive strategies to protect your competitive advantages for as long as possible.

An organization cannot directly control the intensity of rivalry in an industry, but it can benefit from certain strategic actions. Some organizations may seek to intertwine themselves into their customers' business so as to make the customer dependent on them (e.g., Dell computers). Some may adopt strategies of increasing product differentiation to separate themselves from the crowd, raising customers' switching costs by customizing applications or products to build dependency, providing services and repairs for their products, or focusing sales and marketing efforts on areas that have some form of advantage, such as high growth or low fixed costs. We see these efforts frequently in healthcare through the lens of electronic health records.

Consider the highly competitive healthcare marketplace of today. For the last few decades, hospitals have been doing all in their power to maintain and solidify their dominance in the market. Many hospitals, for instance, have bought private practices to provide for a ready self-referral network. This strategy had previously been unsuccessful but is now becoming popular among physicians tired of the increasingly complex healthcare business environment.

Threat of Substitute Products

The availability of substitute products limits the amount of money a company can charge for its product or service. All things being equal, if prices rise, customers will switch to a cheaper competitor to substitute an equivalent product. In reality, the competing options in a market are rarely equivalent. But when they are, the product is referred to as a "commodity" product—in other words, the product is perceived to be the same regardless of where it was purchased. Crude oil is one example of a commodity product. An example from the healthcare industry is generic drugs.

Some products may not be considered equal but have only a limited degree of difference. For example, a consumer may have a preference for a particular brand of gasoline, but if the price for that brand increases more than a few cents per gallon over competitors' prices, the consumer will substitute a lower-priced brand. In the example of generic drugs, some consumers feel loyalty to their personal brand but, in the face of significant changes in reimbursement, will become more accepting of lower-cost options.

Strong brand loyalty, clear product differentiation, and other strategies that create distinction can reduce the threat of substitute products. The ability to substitute is influenced not just by intrinsic product attributes but also by such factors as political constraints and geographic shipping costs. People in the healthcare industry see substitutes frequently, and maintaining product loyalty can be difficult.

Bargaining Power of Suppliers

The power held by raw material, component, subassembly, assembly, transportation, disposal, and other suppliers to companies in an industry directly affects the competitive nature of the industry. The theory of supply and demand suggests that, if there are only a small number of suppliers of a necessary component, prices will rise. Suppliers can hold the corporate buyer "over a barrel."

For example, in the computer industry, microprocessors were once at risk of becoming a commodity item. Retail consumers did not see them or understand them. However, the technology company Intel employed a strategy to change the microprocessor from a commodity item into a branded item. Through a combination of outstanding product development and intense marketing, retail consumers were convinced that having "Intel Inside" made a computer better. Retail customers began to demand Intel processors in the computers they purchased, which in turn put pressure on the original equipment manufacturers (OEMs) to incorporate Intel processors into their computers.

Intel gained significant bargaining power as a supplier to OEMs like IBM and Hewlett-Packard. If OEMs wanted to create a product with an Intel microprocessor, they *had to* buy from Intel. These conditions gave Intel greater power in negotiations over price and terms with the OEMs. As a result, Intel processors became significantly more expensive than competitive processors. Can you think of other computer hardware component parts that have such a demand? Probably not. An OEM can substitute one supplier's motherboard for another supplier's motherboard, because motherboard suppliers have little to no bargaining power. But what about operating systems? Do consumers demand Microsoft operating systems or no-name open-source operating systems? Microsoft has significant bargaining power over the OEMs.

Drug manufacturers have used a similar approach, with direct-to-consumer marketing designed to brand their products. Consumers now approach providers with specific requests for a particular drug, as opposed to the generic substitute, because they have gained familiarity with the branded product and perceive it to be superior. As described earlier, however, this preference will only go so far. If the price goes up significantly, that preference will become less important.

Another category of supplier not found in general business consists of the physicians and surgeons who provide services to healthcare organizations. Most are independent contractors who essentially provide labor to the hospitals. Healthcare organizations must recognize the power of these providers and work to meet their needs through efficient and effective support services.

Bargaining Power of Buyers

The bargaining power of buyers is the opposite of the power of suppliers. If large corporate buyers can shop around for their raw material, components, subassemblies, or other inputs and find lower prices, then these buyers have significant power over their suppliers. Conditions through which industry buyers can gain bargaining power include the following:

- The buyer buys in sufficiently large amounts to be able to demand lower prices.
- The buyer buys in sufficiently large amounts to make the supplier dependent on the purchase.
- The buyer has the ability to easily switch to a different supplier.
- The buyer has the option of dropping the supplier and fulfilling its own need.
- The buyer has the ability to buy a supplier and cut the current supplier out.
- Quality or brand is unimportant to the business.

EXHIBIT 6.3
Analyzing Threat of Entry

Force	Issue*	Impact on Organization†	Implication for Strategy†
Threat of entry (Overall: low–medium)	1. Government regulation requires licensing and accreditation of hospitals to participate in Medicare and Medicaid programs.	Significant time and resources are spent in achieving and maintaining accreditation and licenses.	Must include strategies to address legal issues and other issues related to accreditation.
	2. Technological developments demand regular changes to meet patient and competitive demands.	Significant replacement costs are involved.	Must include strategies to ensure our organization is well positioned technologically to keep competitors from the market.
	3. Competitors in close surrounding communities have higher profit margins due to higher levels of specialty and tertiary care.	We risk appearing "less than" due to lack of specialty care availability. New entrants may consider entry if we are not cutting-edge.	Must include a method to develop an expanded scope of services to better compete with larger competitors and keep them from entering.
	4. Dominant players have the ability to buy smaller players, thus consolidating costs and expanding market share.	Industry consolidation is becoming the norm in healthcare, and it requires significant resources. Our organization may appear vulnerable.	Must include proactive strategies to address industry consolidation (systemization) or a method to compete in a consolidated industry.
	5. Exclusive supplier contracts are in place with major buyers, which currently lock out new suppliers.	We may find ourselves at a competitive disadvantage if suppliers are limited too much.	Must include strategies that allow for evaluation of suppliers on a regular basis to ensure competitive pricing is available so that new entrants see us as competitive.

* Note that the Issue is relative to the *industry*.
† Note that the Impact on Organization and Implication for Strategy are specific to the *company* being studied.

The same rules apply for hospitals and other healthcare organizations. The systemization of healthcare aims largely for efficiency and economies of scale, and it provides an excellent example of the bargaining power of buyers. For example, we seek bids for everything from surgical gowns to hospital beds to multimillion-dollar technologies for patient care. We must have all of these items, and we wish to pay a reasonable price for them.

Consider the time a recent university student was asked during an internship to evaluate the supply of hospital beds, both leased and purchased. Specific bids were received, and the buying power of the local hospital system that uses a large number of beds allowed for a significantly reduced price. Another example involved the contract for security services, which was found to be extremely expensive. Additional bids were sought and millions were saved annually because the company providing the services, not wanting to lose the contract, readily renegotiated a better price.

The bargaining power of buyers is found up and down the value chain, and not just within the hospital or other large entities. It is found in the bed manufacturer's relationship with the steel manufacturer that provides the material for the bed springs. It is found with the supplier of tongue depressors, which purchases wood from those who grow and process wood products. It even encompasses you and me, who purchase healthcare services.

Analyzing the Five Forces

To assess the five forces, the analyst considers each force, one at a time. The analyst identifies all the issues that impact the particular force, how each issue that has been identified affects the company, and what implications each issue has for strategy. Exhibit 6.3 provides an example of an analysis of the threat of entry for hospitals.

Note that "Implication for Strategy" is different from "Strategy." An implication for strategy identifies a broad possibility and allows for future brainstorming of many different strategies that could respond to that possibility. In contrast, identifying a particular strategy here ends the discussion and shuts out other possible strategies that have not yet been considered. For example, Issue 4 in the exhibit has many possible strategic responses. If the issue had instead been addressed with "Buy out a supplier," that strategy would be identified and the search for strategies would be over, eliminating other, maybe better, strategies that could have been developed.

Reference

Porter, M. E. 1980. *Competitive Strategy: Techniques for Analyzing Industries and Competitors.* New York: Free Press.

EXERCISE

Use the blank five forces table to list the issues, impacts, and strategic implications for your project organization.

Five Forces Table

Five Forces	Issue	Impact on Organization	Implication for Strategy
Threat of entry (Overall: low, medium, or high)	1.		
	2.		
	3.		
	4.		
	5.		
Intensity of rivalry (Overall: low, medium, or high)	1.		
	2.		
	3.		
	4.		
	5.		

(continued)

EXERCISE

Five Forces	Issue	Impact on Organization	Implication for Strategy
Threat of substitutes (Overall: low, medium, or high)	1.		
	2.		
	3.		
	4.		
	5.		
Power of suppliers (Overall: low, medium, or high)	1.		
	2.		
	3.		
	4.		
	5.		

Five Forces	Issue	Impact on Organization	Implication for Strategy
Power of buyers (Overall: low, medium, or high)	1.		
	2.		
	3.		
	4.		
	5.		

EXERCISE

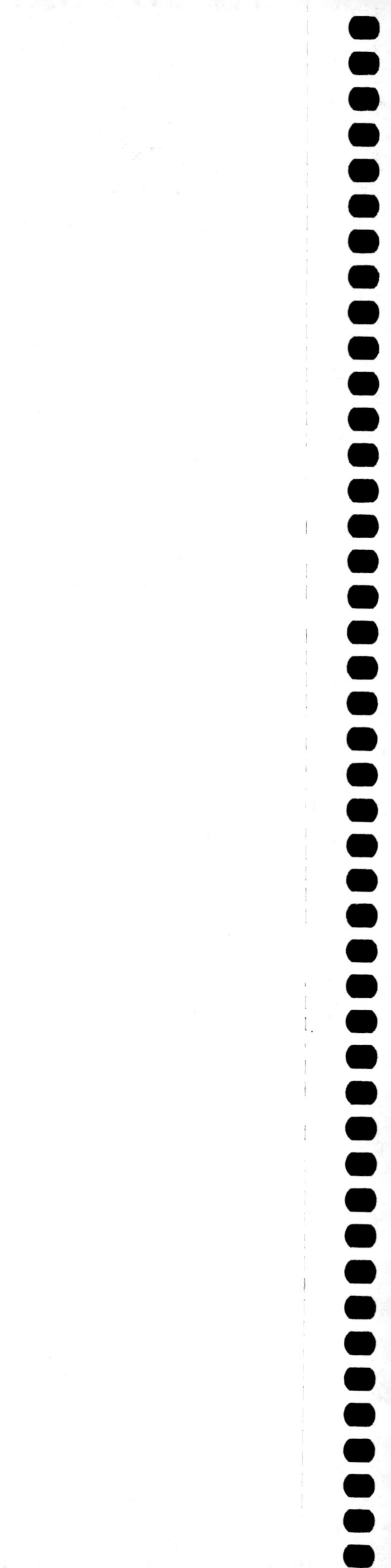

CHAPTER

7

PEST ANALYSIS OF THE ENVIRONMENT

Another tool, the PEST analysis, helps you examine conditions much more broadly than does the five forces analysis. *PEST* stands for *political*, *economic*, *social*, and *technological*—the four perspectives from which the process examines the environment. (Some authors have added the words *environmental* and *legal* to form the acronym *PESTEL*; for our purposes, however, environmental and legal matters fall under the political, because both areas tend to be politically charged and regulated within healthcare.) The purpose of a PEST analysis is to look at the macroenvironment that affects the product you are proposing, the company you are analyzing, or the industry in which it competes.

The timing and success of particular strategies can be influenced positively or negatively by political, economic, social, and technological factors. The strategic analyst studies the macroenvironment both as an input to strategy and as a limiting factor on strategy. Strategic inputs may involve issues identified in an environmental analysis that lead to opportunities for a company (e.g., a huge influx of China's rural population into urban areas, leading to a need for increased retail outlets). Other findings may limit opportunities for a company's strategy (e.g., low disposable income per capita in Zimbabwe, limiting the ability of residents to afford a proposed product). Imagine you are considering building a plastic and reconstructive surgery center in a small, rural Alabama community. A PEST analysis might show that, though there are people in the area with sufficient resources to pay for reconstructive surgery, such people are not the norm; therefore, that area might not be a suitable place for that kind of facility. The environment can be analyzed at multiple levels depending on business need. One could perform a PEST analysis on a single state (California), country (Colombia), trading block (European Union), or region of the world (South America).

For example, a company considering the acquisition of a California business might perform a PEST analysis of the state. The company would want to understand all the political implications of doing business in California. Such implications might include a high minimum wage, an excessive tax structure, state Occupational Safety and Health Administration (OSHA) requirements that exceed federal OSHA requirements, environmental regulations, a legislature less friendly to business, and so on. These factors need to be analyzed and included in the decision of whether to buy the business. Some of these issues will make the cost of doing business higher in California than in other states; as a result, the acquirer would need to adjust its break-even point on the acquisition and develop strategies to compensate. Other PEST factors may help offset the political concerns—for instance, ease of access to new technology partners in Silicon Valley.

EXHIBIT 7.1 Questions to Consider in a PEST Analysis

Political

1. How stable is the political environment you are analyzing?
2. How will government policy influence your ability to do business and make a profit?
3. What is the risk of war, conflict, civil unrest, or trade wars?
4. How favorable are the existing tax laws regarding your industry and, potentially, your business?
5. What is the government's position on financial reporting and corporate transparency?
6. What is the government's economic policy?
7. What impact does religion have on government and law?
8. Does the location belong to international trade agreements?
9. Will tax policy encourage or discourage business? Is it stable?
10. What kind of employment laws are in place?
11. What are the existing environmental regulations, and how are they trending?
12. What is the dominant political ideology?
13. What are the trade restrictions and tariffs?

Economic

1. What are the short-, middle-, and long-term prospects for the economy?
2. What is the average disposable income, and how is income distributed?
3. What are the interest rates?
4. What is the rate of inflation?
5. What employment trends have appeared in recent years?
6. What are the exchange rates?
7. What is the gross domestic product per capita?
8. Is the economy predicted to be in a state of growth, stagnation, or recession?
9. What is the weather trend and impact on work, people, and economics?

Social

1. What are the cultural aspects of the area you are analyzing?
2. What are the roles of men and women in the society?
3. What are the demographic distributions of the population?
4. What are the population growth trends?
5. What is the dominant religion?
6. What are the work ethics and career attitudes of the area?
7. How is education valued?
8. How much time do residents have for leisure?
9. What is the role of the media, and what is the level of freedom of the press?
10. What attitudes exist toward foreign companies and products?
11. How does language affect such things as employment and advertising?
12. What is the influence of tradition, and who are the keepers of tradition?
13. What people are regarded as role models, and what are the ideals?
14. What is the popular view of the environmental impact of industry?
15. What are the major lifestyle trends?

Technological

1. Does the location have available technology infrastructure?
2. Does the location have available technological resources?
3. What is the area's overall research and development investment rate?
4. How advanced is the manufacturing capability?
5. Can products or services be produced more cheaply there due to technology?
6. Is technology available to produce high-quality products and services?
7. Do consumers and businesses take advantage of, and demand, technology?
8. Is technology sufficient to allow for effective distribution systems?
9. Does technology permit consumers the ability to shop suppliers?
10. What is the rate of technological change?
11. How advanced is educational capability?

To perform a PEST analysis, the analyst considers each PEST factor one at a time. The analyst identifies what issues influence each particular factor, how each issue affects the company, and what strategic implications can be drawn from the issues. Exhibit 7.1 lists some of the questions you might consider when performing a PEST analysis.

EXHIBIT 7.2
Social Factor Analysis

PEST Factor	Issue	Impact on Organization	Implication for Strategy
Social	Extended families moving into homes of younger family members	Increased consumer demand for healthcare services due to growing number of older patients	Opportunities to market to the older generation as extended families move in; opportunities to penetrate the geriatric market and expand existing services for older population
	Intolerance developing for immigrants and imported products	Consumers less likely to purchase our product because we are nonlocal in origin	Must address the import-versus-domestic company perception
	Decreasing number of high school graduates entering healthcare programs in the region	Reduced availability of health service professionals	Must develop strategy for increasing availability of professional staff
	Increasing work pressures and decreasing leisure time	Direct impact unclear	Opportunity to develop health-related products and services, such as massage therapy, that may relate to growing needs

Exhibit 7.2 provides an example of an analysis focusing on social aspects. Note again that "Implication for Strategy" is different from "Strategy." An implication for strategy identifies a broad possibility and allows for future brainstorming of many strategies that could respond to that possibility. By contrast, identifying a particular strategy here ends the discussion and shuts out other possible strategies.

Use the PEST table below to list the issues, impacts, and strategic implications for your industry.

PEST	Issue	Impact on Organization	Implication for Strategy
Political	1.		
	2.		
	3.		
	4.		
	5.		
Economic	1.		
	2.		
	3.		
	4.		
	5.		

(continued)

EXERCISE

EXERCISE

PEST	Issue	Impact on Organization	Implication for Strategy
Social	1.		
	2.		
	3.		
	4.		
	5.		
Technological	1.		
	2.		
	3.		
	4.		
	5.		

CHAPTER

8

COMPETITIVE MARKET BENCHMARK ANALYSIS

Understanding the position of competitors in the market is essential for the development of effective business strategy. One way analysts achieve this understanding is through competitive market benchmark analysis. This approach helps analysts identify key factors that differentiate a company from its competition. Benchmarking—that is, establishing goals through comparisons with other organizations' performance—is widely used in healthcare as a quality improvement tool, and it can be extremely helpful in ensuring a competitive advantage over the competition. Analysts are able to use comparisons and differentiation to drive strategy development. For example, consider a company that currently ranks first in market share but sees a competitor quickly rising in the rankings for price, quality, service, and reputation. Benchmark analysis helps the company identify this new competition and decide what to do about it.

To begin a benchmark analysis, analysts need to identify what factors are important in the industry being studied. Each industry has a unique set of critical success factors, key competencies, requirements, and indicators. In most industries, analysts evaluate productivity. In retail sales, for instance, productivity has been measured in sales per square foot, and this measure serves as a key indicator of the efficiency of operations, trends (when measured over time), and competitive position (when compared to other retailers). At healthcare organizations, we evaluate conditions across a number of categories (operations, finance, and so on), and we compare our own organizations with organizations considered to be the best in those specific categories, in or out of healthcare.

Conducting a competitive market benchmark analysis involves a series of steps. First, through research, select the appropriate broad categories for your organization. These categories may include, but are not limited to, the following:

- Product/service categories
- Finance
- Productivity
- Human resources
- Facility

Second, identify the particular factors within those broad categories that are important to your industry. For example, within the finance category, "return on assets" might be important in an industry such as manufacturing, which is highly dependent on equipment. At the same time, "number of accounts 30 to 59 days past due" would likely be much more important in the retail credit industry. Examples of broad categories and key factors common in healthcare are provided in Exhibit 8.1. In conducting your analysis, you can select as many factors as you feel are important.

EXHIBIT 8.1
Categories for Benchmark Analysis

Possible Broad Categories and Key Factors

Product/Service
Expanding markets
Pricing structure
New services and related products
Product/service life cycle
Innovation
Product image/reputation
Perceived quality

Finance
Operating ratios
Average length of stay
Collection rate
Gross margin ratio
Return on equity
Return on assets
Debt-to-equity ratio

Productivity
Market share
Growth percentage
Corporate image
Patient loyalty
Revenue per unit
Advertising/marketing

Human Resources
Average number of employees
Annual revenue per employee
Annual compensation per employee
Flexibility of organizational structure
Ability to attract and retain the best people

Facility
Size of existing facilities
Age of existing facilities
Size of emergency department
Trauma center
Age of administration space
Room for expansion

In identifying factors, analysts sometimes fall into conceptual traps such as failure to think in the big picture or failure to move from the present to the future tense. Consider the US automotive industry in the 1960s. The industry failed to foresee the oil crisis of the 1970s, the growth of the Japanese automotive industry, and the trend of increasing consumer sensitivity to price and quality. Looking back, one might wonder how analysts would miss those issues. This example provides a clear picture of the need to think broadly and consider future possibilities. American auto industry analysts could have, and in retrospect *should* have, identified those issues and enabled the US industry to stop the Japanese industry in its tracks. Healthcare is different from the auto industry, but the key points still apply. Consider the rapidly evolving healthcare system in the United Sates. People have long acknowledged that some type of reform is necessary, but few have agreed on how to approach it. Can you consider the big picture to address the healthcare needs in your community and develop a strategy to ensure the competitive viability of your organization well into the future?

As the third step, identify the competition in your area, and obtain their information for each key factor you have identified. Laying the results out in a table allows for easier presentation and quick grasp of the issues. Consider adding an "industry average" column to compare your organization to the averages. You can choose from a number of methods for finding how the competitors compare. Common methods include numeric data reporting, forced ranking (in which competitors are assigned ranks from best to worst), scoring (on a point scale of 1 to 5 for each factor, for instance), and selecting "yes" or "no" for key items. Examples of these approaches are presented in Exhibits 8.2 through 8.5.

EXHIBIT 8.2
Analysis Example Using Yes/No

Product/Service	Our Hospital	Alpha Hospital	Beta Hospital	Omega Hospital	Industry
Practice network	YES	NO	NO	YES	Yes
Trauma center	YES	NO	NO	YES	NO
Cancer center	YES	YES	NO	NO	NO
Emergency department	YES	NO	YES	YES	YES

EXHIBIT 8.3
Analysis Example Using Scoring Scale

Human Resources	Our Hospital	Alpha Hospital	Beta Hospital	Omega Hospital	Industry
Overall quality rating	1	2	2	5	3
Retention	2	1	2	5	2
Flexibility	1	4	2	5	3
Onboarding and training	1	4	3	5	3

1 = superior; 5 = poor

EXHIBIT 8.4
Analysis Example Using Numeric Data Reporting

Finance	Our Hospital	Alpha Hospital	Beta Hospital	Omega Hospital	Industry
Liquidity ratio	2.18	1.95	.98	2.02	2.11
Long-term debt to assets	.25	48	67	33	.21
Age-of-plant ratio	9.49	7.80	8.21	5.72	10.31
Average days in accounts receivable	48	59	62	54	49

EXHIBIT 8.5
Analysis Example Using Forced Ranking

Productivity	Our Hospital	Alpha Hospital	Beta Hospital	Omega Hospital	Median
Market share	1	2	3	4	2.5
Adjusted operating revenue	2	4	3	1	2.5
Revenue per provider	2	4	1	3	2.5
Patient loyalty	1	3	2	4	2.5

1 = superior; 5 = poor

Fourth, extract meaning from the data. Ask questions like, "Why is it so?" "Who is the best of the best and why?" "What trends are visible?" "Given this same data, what are the competitors likely to do?" In subsequent chapters, we will look at strengths, weaknesses, opportunities, and threats (SWOT). Findings from the competitive market benchmark analysis will provide you with some of the information necessary to complete the SWOT analysis.

Again, remember to think broadly. Your competition includes anything that could compete with your organization, not just your peer group. For example, movie theaters compete with other theaters directly, but they also compete indirectly with cable TV, video rentals, electronic games, websites, restaurants, live music venues, Broadway-style theater, and circuses, to name a few. In healthcare, alternative providers are but one category of potential competitors.

When a benchmark analysis contains both financial and nonfinancial information, it is often called a balanced scorecard. The word *balanced* reflects the fact that many companies in the past only measured themselves and their competitors based on financial data. The inclusion of a broad range of categories, from corporate culture to technical innovation, gives the strategic analyst a deeper insight into the company under study, the competitors, and the industry. This insight will likely lead to a more effective strategy.

Conduct a competitive market benchmark analysis for your industry. Follow the steps below.

EXERCISE

Competitive Market Benchmark Analysis of the ______________________________ Industry

1. Identify the key broad categories for your industry.

   1.

   2.

   3.

   4.

   5.

(continued)

EXERCISE

2. Within those categories, identify the key factors for your industry. Consider your company, identify your competitors, and complete the table using one of the approaches identified in this chapter.

Category	Your Company	Competitor 1	Competitor 2	Competitor 3	Industry
1.					
a.					
b.					
c.					
d.					
e.					
f.					
g.					
2.					
a.					
b.					
c.					
d.					
e.					
f.					
g.					

Category	Your Company	Competitor 1	Competitor 2	Competitor 3	Industry
3.					
a.					
b.					
c.					
d.					
e.					
f.					
g.					
4.					
a.					
b.					
c.					
d.					
e.					
f.					
g.					

(continued)

EXERCISE

Category	Your Company	Competitor 1	Competitor 2	Competitor 3	Industry
5.					
a.					
b.					
c.					
d.					
e.					
f.					
g.					

3. List the implications for your company's strategy.

1.

2.

3.

4.

5.

6.

7.

8.

9.

10.

CHAPTER

9

SWOT: EXTERNAL OPPORTUNITIES AND THREATS

An Introduction to SWOT

Analysis of an organization's strengths, weaknesses, opportunities, and threats is commonly called SWOT analysis. SWOT brings together analyses from the previous chapters and starts to form a cohesive assessment of the company. SWOT does not identify particular strategies but rather identifies issues that may later need to be strategically addressed. Specific consideration is given to critical success factors in the firm's industry. The SWOT categories are examined in two dimensions, covering internal and external issues, as shown in Exhibit 9.1.

Internally, every organization has both strengths and weaknesses. As a prelude to developing strategy, the analyst must understand what these strengths and weaknesses are, particularly in relation to the industry's critical success factors. An aggressive strategy for research and development (R&D) and new product introduction might not be appropriate for a company that is weak in the area of engineering, R&D, or manufacturing capability. In healthcare, for example, a hospital system delivering direct patient care may not consider technology transfer itself, based on its research activities, but may want to partner with others more experienced in that area. A more fundamental strategy might be to strengthen areas of weakness before venturing into uncharted waters. Opportunities and threats, described in greater detail later in this chapter, are regarded as the external SWOT factors.

A company's SWOT analysis is typically depicted in a four-block matrix as shown in Exhibit 9.2. An alternative display used by some strategists involves listing the organization along with top competitors in the area or region, side by side, as shown in Exhibit 9.3. The purpose of this format is to more easily compare the SWOT components of one company to its competitors in a simple display.

The SWOT analysis will serve as the basis for two lines of analysis that we will explore in the chapters ahead. The first line will involve developing an internal factor evaluation (IFE) and an external factor evaluation (EFE), leading to an internal–external (I/E) matrix

EXHIBIT 9.1
Dimensions of SWOT Analysis

Internal:	Strengths	Weaknesses
External:	Opportunities	Threats

EXHIBIT 9.2
SWOT Analysis Matrix

Company Name

Strengths	Weaknesses
Opportunities	Threats

EXHIBIT 9.3
Company Grid for SWOT Analysis with Competitors

	Your Company	Competitor 1	Competitor 2	Competitor 3
Strengths	1.	1.	1.	1.
	2.	2.	2.	2.
	3.	3.	3.	3.
	4.	4.	4.	4.
	5.	5.	5.	5.
	6.	6.	6.	6.
	7.	7.	7.	7.
	8.	8.	8.	8.
	9.	9.	9.	9.
	10.	10.	10.	10.
Weaknesses	1.	1.	1.	1.
	2.	2.	2.	2.
	3.	3.	3.	3.
	4.	4.	4.	4.
	5.	5.	5.	5.
	6.	6.	6.	6.
	7.	7.	7.	7.
	8.	8.	8.	8.
	9.	9.	9.	9.
	10.	10.	10.	10.
Opportunities	1.	1.	1.	1.
	2.	2.	2.	2.
	3.	3.	3.	3.
	4.	4.	4.	4.
	5.	5.	5.	5.
	6.	6.	6.	6.
	7.	7.	7.	7.
	8.	8.	8.	8.
	9.	9.	9.	9.
	10.	10.	10.	10.

(continued)

EXHIBIT 9.3 Company Grid for SWOT Analysis with Competitors (continued)

	Your Company	Competitor 1	Competitor 2	Competitor 3
Threats	1.	1.	1.	1.
	2.	2.	2.	2.
	3.	3.	3.	3.
	4.	4.	4.	4.
	5.	5.	5.	5.
	6.	6.	6.	6.
	7.	7.	7.	7.
	8.	8.	8.	8.
	9.	9.	9.	9.
	10.	10.	10.	10.

that suggests broad strategic directions. In the second line of analysis, SWOT will form the basis of a TOWS (*SWOT* written backward) matrix that will be used to develop specific strategies. See Exhibit 9.4.

SWOT: The External Analysis

Most strategy texts instruct the analyst to complete all four SWOT boxes at one time. This text, however, separates the internal and external components and addresses them separately. Doing so allows the strategist to focus on the external issues first and to draw upon the previous analyses that were primarily external in focus. We will examine the internal SWOT factors in Chapter 17, after having had an opportunity to perform additional analyses of the inner workings of the company.

The external factors account for SWOT's *O* and *T*—the opportunities and the threats. An opportunity can be thought of as any market possibility for which your organization can take action and make a positive impact. Such impacts could include organizational growth, market share increase, potential entry into new markets, increased profits, chances to exploit competitors' weaknesses, or any other positive outcome. Today in

EXHIBIT 9.4 Where Is SWOT Leading?

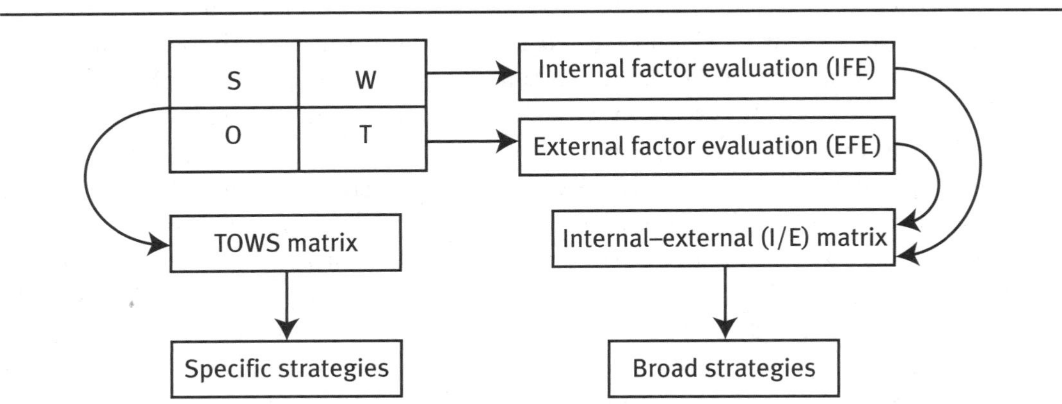

EXHIBIT 9.5
Examples of a Company's External Opportunities and Threats

Opportunities	Threats
1. Expansion of existing services	1. Multiple competitors
2. Additional locations	2. Emergency department overcrowding
3. Greater exposure and branding	3. Power of suppliers
4. Addition of trauma center	4. Recent lawsuits
5. Purchasing additional practices	5. Low socioeconomic status
6. Expansion into surrounding counties	6. Transient market
7. Government contracts	7. Dependence on suppliers
8. Residency programs/teaching	8. Difficulty recruiting providers
9. Expansion of ancillary services	9. Changes in reimbursement
10. Demographic changes	10. Decrease in population

healthcare, for instance, the systemization of hospitals is becoming commonplace, and it represents an opportunity for well-positioned organizations to grow.

A threat can be defined as any possibility for your company to be negatively affected by an external action of the market or of a competitor. Threats represent negative impacts on your company's profitability and competitive well-being. Negative impacts could involve such things as competitor plans to introduce new technology or services to attract your current customer base, economic forces, the potential of a hostile takeover, the chance of a new entrant into your market, or looming price wars. On the converse of the systemization example presented above, larger hospitals coming into a market and buying up smaller competitors to form systems may be seen as a threat.

When you begin your SWOT analysis, first focus on the external factors that could, either now or in the future, affect your organization. Consider the critical success factors that pertain to the external environment. Where does this information come from? It should draw upon your research about the organization in particular, the industry, and the external environment in general. You have previously assessed these issues to develop your industry map, five forces analysis, PEST analysis, and competitive benchmark analysis. Review those analyses and identify the issues that could become competitive threats against your organization or could create competitive opportunities for your organization. Typically, you should identify about ten opportunities and ten threats. Note that you are not proposing strategies or solutions at this time. You are identifying critical issues that will need to be addressed in subsequent strategy development sections.

You need to think broadly here. Consider the local hospitals of the 1980s. They were the facilities sought by all and trusted for their healthcare, much like family physicians. As we are aware, times have changed, and the delivery of healthcare changed along with it; we must constantly revisit our SWOT analysis to ensure that we are doing things right and doing the right things.

Though some threats may seem remote, they still may be worth addressing. In the case of oil prices, for example, the potential for a rise in prices could have been reflected in the economic section of an automotive company's PEST analysis. Similarly, the threat of war or oil embargos could have been identified in the political section. These issues could then have been transferred directly into the SWOT analysis. You should carefully examine your previous analyses to identify issues for the external section of SWOT. Exhibit 9.5 provides a hypothetical example for a small healthcare organization.

Complete the external portion of the SWOT analysis for your project organization in the space provided. Be sure to review your previous analyses and consider the critical success factors in the industry. What are the implications for strategy? The issues you identify in this exercise will be used to complete the EFE in the next chapter and later will be transferred into the TOWS strategy development chart in Chapter 24.

EXERCISE

(SW)OT Analysis of ______________________________

External:	**Opportunities**	**Threats**
	1.	1.
	2.	2.
	3.	3.
	4.	4.
	5.	5.
	6.	6.
	7.	7.
	8.	8.
	9.	9.
	10.	10.

EXERCISE

Implications for Strategy:

1.

2.

3.

4.

5.

6.

7.

8.

9.

10.

CHAPTER

10

EXTERNAL FACTOR EVALUATION

An external factor evaluation (EFE) organizes and evaluates the *OT* section—opportunities and threats—of SWOT. The EFE produces a numeric score that reflects the gravity of each issue combined with management's current response to it. The resulting score will correspond to certain standard strategies that will be discussed in Chapter 19.

As a starting point, consider that not every item you identified in the *OT* section of your SWOT analysis is of equal threat or has equal opportunity value. Some distinction needs to be made between the "great" opportunities and the "could be" opportunities. To help make these distinctions, review a list of each opportunity and threat. The sample list from the previous chapter is repeated in Exhibit 10.1.

EXHIBIT 10.1 Examples of External Opportunities and Threats

Opportunities
1. Expansion of existing services
2. Additional locations
3. Greater exposure and branding
4. Addition of trauma center
5. Purchasing additional practices
6. Expansion into surrounding counties
7. Government contracts
8. Residency programs/teaching
9. Expansion of ancillary services
10. Demographic changes

Threats
1. Multiple competitors
2. Emergency department overcrowding
3. Power of suppliers
4. Recent lawsuits
5. Low socioeconomic status
6. Transient market
7. Dependence on suppliers
8. Difficulty recruiting providers
9. Changes in reimbursement
10. Decrease in population

EXHIBIT 10.2
Weighting of Opportunities and Threats

Opportunities	Weight
1. Expansion of existing services	0.050
2. Additional locations	0.100
3. Greater exposure and branding	0.050
4. Addition of trauma center	0.025
5. Purchasing additional practices	0.025
6. Expansion into surrounding counties	0.075
7. Government contracts	0.025
8. Residency programs/teaching	0.025
9. Expansion of ancillary services	0.050
10. Demographic changes	0.050

Threats	Weight
1. Multiple competitors	0.100
2. Emergency department overcrowding	0.100
3. Power of suppliers	0.025
4. Recent lawsuits	0.025
5. Low socioeconomic status	0.050
6. Transient market	0.075
7. Dependence on suppliers	0.025
8. Difficulty recruiting providers	0.075
9. Changes in reimbursement	0.025
10. Decrease in population	0.025
Total weight:	1.00

Now, the strategist evaluates each opportunity and threat and applies a weighting system. The total weight is 1.00 when all of the weights have been applied and added. Each individual factor, therefore, receives some portion of 1.00. The size of that portion reflects the strategist's subjective evaluation of how important each external factor is to successful competition within the industry. The more important the factor, the higher is the weight assigned. Building on the previous example, Exhibit 10.2 shows the weights assigned to individual opportunities and threats. The total of 1.00 is the sum of the whole column, including both opportunities and threats.

The table shows that the threat related to emergency department overcrowding is important; it has been deemed by the strategist to be much more significant than the threat posed by recent lawsuits or the opportunity of obtaining more government contracts. Note that there is no one "correct" weight for any factor. The accuracy of the analysis rests squarely on the shoulders of the strategist. For that reason, significant research and a clear understanding of the company and industry are vital to the process.

Once weights have been assigned, the strategist next focuses on management's response to each issue. The relevant question is, "How well does management *currently* respond to this factor?" The focus is on management's current response—not on its potential future response or its responses in the past. Management's response is rated on a scale of 1 to 4 as follows:

4 = Current response is superior.
3 = Current response is above average.
2 = Current response is average.
1 = Current response is poor.

The rating for management's response to each factor is once again subjective on the part of the strategist, and once again it should be based on research. These ratings are not added up, so there are no constraints on how the numbers may be distributed. Once the current response ratings have been applied, the rating for each particular factor is multiplied by that factor's weight; the resulting number is a weighted score for the factor. Exhibit 10.3 continues the example from previous exhibits.

The EFE analysis yields a total score when the column of individual scores is summed. This total score can be used to complete an internal–external (I/E) matrix,

EXHIBIT 10.3
EFE Total Score

EFE Analysis

Opportunities	Weight*	Rating†	Score
1. Expansion of existing services	0.050	4	0.2
2. Additional locations	0.100	2	0.2
3. Greater exposure and branding	0.050	2	0.1
4. Addition of trauma center	0.025	1	0.025
5. Purchasing additional practices	0.025	2	0.05
6. Expansion into surrounding counties	0.075	2	0.15
7. Government contracts	0.025	3	0.075
8. Residency programs/teaching	0.025	2	0.05
9. Expansion of ancillary services	0.050	2	0.1
10. Demographic changes	0.050	2	0.1

Threats	Weight	Rating	Score
1. Multiple competitors	0.100	2	0.2
2. Emergency department overcrowding	0.100	3	0.3
3. Power of suppliers	0.025	2	0.05
4. Recent lawsuits	0.025	2	0.05
5. Low socioeconomic status	0.050	3	0.15
6. Transient market	0.075	1	0.075
7. Dependence on suppliers	0.025	3	0.075
8. Difficulty recruiting providers	0.075	3	0.225
9. Changes in reimbursement	0.025	2	0.05
10. Decrease in population	0.025	2	0.05
Total weight:	1.00	**Total score:**	2.275

* Weight is industry specific.
† Rating is organization specific.

which in turn corresponds to a standard table of strategies linked to particular I/E scores. For now, we will not concern ourselves with the general strategies, but we will return to the subject and to the EFE rating score later. We will address the *SW* factors of SWOT and the I/E matrix in later chapters as well.

Review your previous analyses and develop an EFE analysis for your project organization.

EXERCISE

EFE Analysis of ______________________________

Opportunities	Weight	Rating	Score
1.			
2.			
3.			
4.			
5.			
6.			
7.			
8.			
9.			
10.			

(continued)

EXERCISE

Threats	Weight	Rating	Score
1.			
2.			
3.			
4.			
5.			
6.			
7.			
8.			
9.			
10.			

Total weight: ____________ **Total score:** ____________

Rating scale:

4 = Current response is superior.
3 = Current response is above average.
2 = Current response is average.
1 = Current response is poor.

PART

FOCUSED ANALYSIS

CHAPTER

11

FINANCIAL STATEMENT AND RATIO ANALYSIS

Shifting from broad analysis to focused analysis, you will need to conduct a careful review of your company's financial statements. A firm's financial statements consist of three main sections: the balance sheet, the income statement, and the statement of cash flows. In addition, you should review other associated documents, such as a public company's 10-K.

Financial Ratio Analysis

The analysis of an organization's financial ratios combines an internal analysis of the firm's finances with an external comparison of the same factors. The financial data you choose to look at depends on the particular organization and the specific industry. Financial ratios can be grouped into several broad categories—liquidity, leverage, activity, profitability, growth, and valuation—and the analyst should include at least two or three relevant ratios for each. Exhibit 11.1 lists some ratios and their methods of calculation.

EXHIBIT 11.1 Financial Ratio Analysis

Ratio	Formula	What It Tells You	Positive Trend	Comparators
LIQUIDITY RATIOS				
Current ratio	Current assets / Current liabilities	Ability to pay short-term debts	Higher	Peer group, historical average, rule of thumb (>2)
Quick ratio (acid test)	(Cash + Marketable securities + Receivables) / Current liabilities	Financial solvency when inventory is not easily liquidated	Higher	Peer group, historical average, rule of thumb (>1)
Cash from operations ratio	Cash from operations (a.k.a. operating cash flow) / Current liabilities	Whether firm is generating enough cash to cover current operations	Higher	Peer group, historical average, rule of thumb (>40%)
Days cash on hand	(Cash + Marketable securities + Long-term investments) / ((Operating expense – Depreciation and amortization) / 365)	Cash available to pay *x* number of days, average cash outflow	Higher	Peer group, historical average
LEVERAGE RATIOS				
Debt-to-total-assets ratio	Total liabilities / Total assets	Percent of total assets being funded by creditors	Lower	Peer group, historical average
Debt-to-equity ratio	Total liabilities / Total equity (or net assets for nonprofits)	Percent of total assets being funded by firm's owners	Lower	Peer group, historical average

(continued)

EXHIBIT 11.1
Financial Ratio Analysis (continued)

Ratio	Formula	What It Tells You	Positive Trend	Comparators
Long-term debt-to-equity ratio	Long-term liabilities / Total equity (or net assets for nonprofits)	Amount of long-term debt a firm has compared to equity	Lower	Peer group, historical average
Times interest earned ratio	Earnings before interest and taxes (a.k.a. EBIT) / Interest expense	How easily a firm can pay interest due on outstanding debt	Higher	Peer group, historical average
ACTIVITY RATIOS				
Total asset turnover ratio	Total revenue (a.k.a. sales) / Total assets	Amount of total revenue per dollar of total assets	Higher	Peer group, historical average
Fixed asset turnover	Total revenue (a.k.a. sales) / Fixed assets	Firm's ability to effectively utilize fixed assets	Higher	Peer group, historical average
Inventory turnover	Total revenue (a.k.a. sales) / Inventory	How long sales inventory waits to be sold	Lower	Peer group, historical average
Average collection period	Receivables / Total revenue (a.k.a. sales) / 365	How long it takes to collect monies due	Lower	Peer group, historical average
Age-of-plant ratio	Accumulated depreciation / Depreciation expense	How old the plant and equipment are; newer is better	Lower	Peer group, historical average
PROFITABILITY RATIOS				
Revenue per adjusted discharge	Operating revenue / (Gross patient revenue / Gross inpatient revenue) × Total discharges	Operating revenue generated from patient care services	Higher	Peer group, historical average
Operating expense per adjusted discharge	Total operating expense / (Gross patient revenue / Gross inpatient revenue) × Total discharges	Expense associated with patient care services	Lower	Peer group, historical average
Salary and benefits as a percentage of operating expense	Salary and benefit expense / Total operating expense	Employee expenses as a percentage of total expenses	Lower	Peer group, historical average
Return on assets (ROA)	Net income (profit) / Total assets	Management's ability to earn a return on each dollar of assets	Higher	Peer group, historical average, economic comparison (avg. weighted cost of capital)
Return on total assets	Excess of revenues over expenses / Total assets	In nonprofit organizations, management's ability to earn a return on each dollar of assets	Higher	Peer group, historical average, economic comparison (avg. weighted cost of capital)
Return on equity (ROE)	Net income (profit) / Shareholders' equity	Rate of return on stockholders' investment	Higher	Peer group, historical average
Return on net assets	Excess of revenues over expenses / Net assets	In nonprofit organizations, rate of return in net assets	Higher	Peer group, historical average
Gross profit margin	Net sales – Cost of goods sold / Net sales	Gross profit margin	Higher	Peer group, historical average
Net profit margin	Net income (profit) / Sales revenue	The amount of net profit as a percentage of sales	Higher	Peer group, historical average

EXHIBIT 11.1
Financial Ratio Analysis (continued)

Ratio	Formula	What It Tells You	Positive Trend	Comparators
Operating margin	Earnings before interest and taxes (from operations) / Net sales	Operating profit margin	Higher	Peer group, historical average
Cash flow margin	Income before depreciation, interest, taxes	Income including nonoperation sources	Higher	Peer group, historical average
Return on capital employed	Earnings before interest and taxes / Total assets – Current liabilities	The efficiency with which capital is employed	Higher	Peer group, historical average
GROWTH RATIOS				
Revenue increase	This year's revenue / Last year's revenue	Percentage increase in revenue year over year	Higher	Peer group, historical average
Earnings per share (EPS)	Net income – Preferred stock dividends / Average outstanding shares	The amount of profit per share of stock	Higher	Peer group, historical average
Dividends payout ratio	Dividends per common share of stock / Earnings per share	The portion of a company's profit paid relative to each common share of stock	Varies	Peer group, historical average
VALUATION RATIOS (FOR PUBLICLY TRADED COMPANIES)				
P/E ratio	Price per share / Earnings per share	How much investors are willing to pay per dollar of earnings	Higher	Peer group, historical average
Dividend yield	Dividends per share / Price per share	Dividend payout as a percentage of stock price	Varies	Peer group, historical average
Dividend payout	Annual dividends per share / After-tax earnings per share	Dividend payout as a percentage of profit	Varies	Peer group, historical average
Cash flow per share	After-tax profits + Depreciation / Number of common shares outstanding	Amount of cash per share of stock	Higher	Peer group, historical average
Price-to-book ratio	Price per share / Total assets – (Intangible assets and liabilities)	Compares a firm's market value to its book value	Higher	Peer group, historical average
PEG ratio	P/E ratio / Annual earnings per share growth	A stock's value while taking the company's earnings growth into consideration	Higher	Peer group, historical average
Return on net worth	Net income / Net worth	Profit as related to the firm's net worth	Higher	Peer group, historical average

Source: Adapted from Gapenski (2011); McArthur (2014); National Association of Certified Valuators and Analysts (2012); Pagach (2014); and Zelman, McCue, and Glick (2009).

The internal financial ratio analysis is concerned with both the current state of the organization and the trend. Knowing that the organization is at "point X" is important to the strategist; even more important, however, is observing a trend and predicting where that trend will lead without intervention. To carry out this kind of observation, the analyst needs to assemble three to five consecutive years of data. Exhibit 11.2 shows a sample grid for completing this analysis. The ratios can be selected from the list in Exhibit 11.1. Once the data has been recorded and reviewed, the analyst should create a list of implications for strategy.

Simply looking at the organization's own financial ratios, however, does not tell an analyst all there is to know. The data needs to be compared to some reference point. Standards exist for every financial ratio, but in competitive analysis and strategy development,

EXHIBIT 11.2
Sample Grid for Trend Analysis

Financial Ratio Data for Company X

	Ratio	Year 1	Year 2	+/–	Year 3	+/–
Liquidity						
Leverage						
Activity						
Profitability						
Growth						
Valuation						

EXHIBIT 11.3
Competitive Financial Ratio Data Chart

Competitive Financial Ratio Data for Company X (as of ______________________)

	Ratio	Our Firm	Competitor 1	+/–	Competitor 2	+/–	Competitor 3	+/–	Peer Group/ Industry	+/–
Liquidity										
Leverage										
Activity										
Profitability										
Growth										
Valuation										

the most relevant comparisons are to the firm's competitors, and then to the industry within which the firm competes. Every industry has its own norms.

For example, a financial analyst may determine that a firm has an extremely high debt-to-equity ratio simply by looking at the numbers. However, the strategist would also like to know how highly leveraged the firm's competitors are, and what the norm is for the particular industry. Exhibit 11.3 shows a grid on which that information can be recorded and analyzed. Again, the analyst should list any implications for strategy that result from the analysis.

An even more powerful tool combines the previous approaches and looks at competitors using five years of financial data, thus allowing the analyst to identify trends for the competitors. The strategist would like to identify deteriorating or improving competitor conditions. Emerging competitor weaknesses can be exploited, and emerging competitor strengths can be defended against. Improving or degrading competitor trends can also be a warning sign for a firm's own vulnerability. To conduct a thorough study, the analyst should complete one five-year financial ratio data chart (see Exhibit 11.2) for each competitor and list the implications for strategy.

References

Gapenski, L. C. 2011. "Online Appendix A: Financial Analysis Ratios." *Healthcare Finance: An Introduction to Accounting and Financial Management*, 5th ed. Book companion. Published November 16. www.ache.org/pubs/hap_companion/gapenski_finance5/HF5Online%20Appendix%20A.pdf.

McArthur, D. N. 2014. "A Summary of Key Financial Ratios: How They Are Calculated and What They Show." Accessed November 2. http://research.uvu.edu/management/mcarthur/Boilerplate/FinanceRatios.pdf.

National Association of Certified Valuators and Analysts. 2012. "Financial Statement Analysis & Calculation of Financial Ratios." Accessed November 2, 2014. http://edu.nacva.com/preread/2012BVTC/2012v1_FTT_Chapter_Two.pdf.

Pagach, D. 2014. "FSA Note: Summary of Financial Ratio Calculations." Accessed November 2. www4.ncsu.edu/~acdon/Note%20on%20Financial%20Ratio%20Formula.pdf.

Zelman, W. N., M. J. McCue, and N. D. Glick. 2009. *Financial Management of Health Care Organizations: An Introduction to Fundamental Tools, Concepts, and Applications.* Hoboken, NJ: Wiley.

EXERCISE

In the spaces provided, complete a financial ratio analysis for your organization, a competitive financial ratio data chart for your competitors, and a financial ratio analysis for each competitor. List the implications for strategy.

Financial Ratio Data for ______________________

	Ratio	Year 1	Year 2	+/–	Year 3	+/–
Liquidity						
Leverage						
Activity						
Profitability						
Growth						
Valuation						

Implications for Strategy from Ratio Comparison:

1.

2.

3.

4.

5.

6.

7.

8.

9.

10.

EXERCISE

Competitive Financial Ratio Data for ____________________

	Ratio	Our Firm	Competitor 1	+/–	Competitor 2	+/–	Competitor 3	+/–	Peer Group/Industry	+/–
Liquidity										
Leverage										
Activity										
Profitability										
Growth										
Valuation										

EXERCISE

Implications for Strategy from Competitive Financial Data:

1.

2.

3.

4.

5.

6.

7.

8.

9.

10.

EXERCISE

Financial Ratio Data for Competitor ______________________

	Ratio	Year 1	Year 2	+/–	Year 3	+/–
Liquidity						
Leverage						
Activity						
Profitability						
Growth						
Valuation						

EXERCISE

Financial Ratio Data for Competitor ______________________

	Ratio	Year 1	Year 2	+/–	Year 3	+/–
Liquidity						
Leverage						
Activity						
Profitability						
Growth						
Valuation						

EXERCISE

Financial Ratio Data for Competitor ______________________

	Ratio	Year 1	Year 2	+/–	Year 3	+/–
Liquidity						
Leverage						
Activity						
Profitability						
Growth						
Valuation						

EXERCISE

Implications for Strategy from Competitors' Data:

1.

2.

3.

4.

5.

6.

7.

8.

9.

10.

CHAPTER

12

BOSTON CONSULTING GROUP MATRIX

During the 1970s, the Boston Consulting Group (BCG 1973) developed an approach to strategic analysis that compares a firm's market share to the anticipated growth of its market in the next five years. The BCG matrix, as the approach became known, is usually used to analyze corporations with multiple divisions or business units. However, it can also be used to analyze a company with only one unit, or even to analyze individual product offerings. Because of its flexibility in this area, the BCG matrix is often called a "portfolio analysis tool." By placing market growth rate on the vertical axis and relative market share on the horizontal axis, a four-block matrix can be developed, as shown in Exhibit 12.1.

Once the firm's business units are positioned on the BCG matrix, strategies are developed based on the units' relative positions. The four quadrants of the matrix, derived by categorizing the two variables into "high" and "low" areas, allow the units to be grouped into four categories: "stars," "question marks," "cash cows," and "dogs" (see Exhibit 12.2). The idea behind the arrangement is that the higher the market growth rate, the more cash is needed from the firm to stay competitive and grow. At the same time, the higher the firm's market share, the more cash can be generated. The cash generated by the high "cash generation" divisions can be used to fund the high "cash consumption" divisions.

If mathematical precision is desired, a quantitative scale can be placed on each axis. For example, if the analyst anticipates that over the next five years the market will grow 30 percent, then the vertical axis can be divided into 5 percent increments, from 0 to 30, and the division's anticipated growth rate can be plotted against it. The division's growth

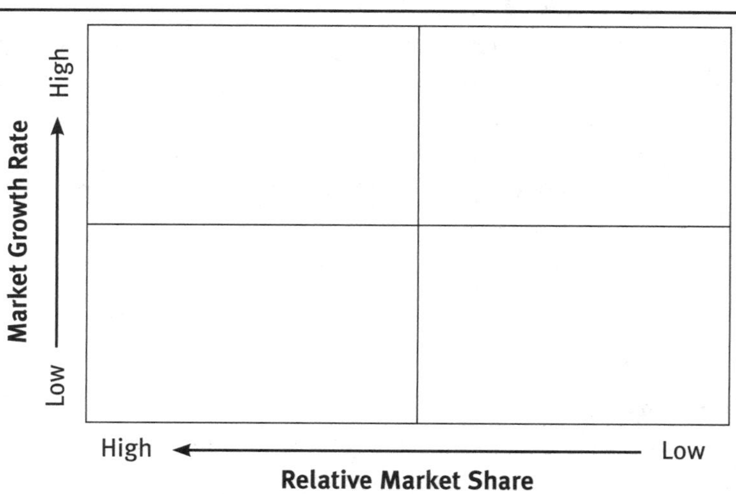

EXHIBIT 12.1 Boston Consulting Group Matrix

EXHIBIT 12.2 Four Quadrants of the BCG Matrix

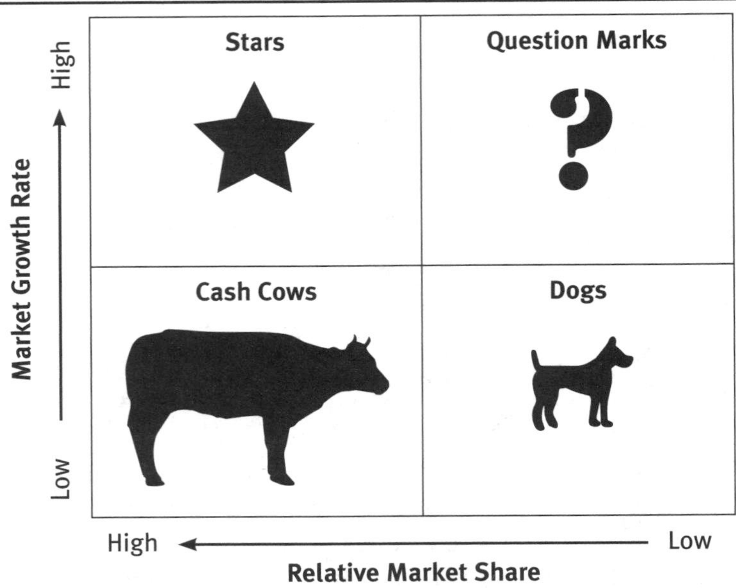

rate would be presented as the division exists today, before any strategic intervention. The market share axis would be shown as a logarithmic scale. This scale would indicate the market share of a division relative to the market share of the largest competitor in its market. For example, Company A may have a 5 percent market share, and the leading competitor, Company B, may have a 20 percent market share. Company A's market share relative to Company B's market share is 25 percent, or .25×. Alternatively, if Company A has a 20 percent market share and Company B has a 5 percent market share, Company A's market share relative to Company B's is 400 percent, or 4.0×.

The ideal movement for a company, division, or product is to move from dog to question mark to star to cash cow. A dysfunctional movement would go in the reverse direction. New products often start in the question mark box. They are introduced into what is anticipated to be a high-growth market but have not generated much cash yet. Time will tell if they move into the star box or the dog box.

A health-related example can be seen in the eye care industry, in the optical dispensary that sells specific products to consumers. Imagine a provider seeks to increase sales in sports vision, which is currently in the dog category. The provider sees a specific need in the community, due to recent sports-related ocular injuries, and starts to educate the public on the need to wear sports eyewear. A combined marketing approach helps move sports vision from dog to question mark, and the unit then shows movement into the star category.

The following sections examine dogs, question marks, stars, and cash cows in greater detail.

Dogs

Dogs are divisions that are not doing well. They have low market share in markets that have low growth. Generally, they tend to neither draw much cash from the parent company nor generate much cash—although sometimes they will require a corporation's cash in order to remain in business. At best, dogs are not adding significant value; at worst, they are drawing off cash and management's time and attention. Therefore, the typical strategies for dogs seek to turn them around and move them toward the question mark box, to divest them, or to shut them down. However, a firm may have strategic reasons for keeping a dog. In the eyewear example above, a niche exists for sports protection; even if positive movement is not seen, the firm may be wise to continue to offer products in, although not focus on, this category.

Question Marks

Question marks are divisions that have low market share in markets that are growing. Because the market is growing, question marks tend to require cash for continued competition. Rather than being net cash generators, question marks tend to draw off a corporation's cash. In these cases, the strategic approach is not clear—hence the term *question mark*. If the strategist sees potential to grow the division's market share and move the division into the star box, strategies may include product development, market penetration, market development, and other growth strategies. If the analyst does not see the potential to improve the division, or if the company does not have the cash to invest in the unit, divestiture may be an option.

Stars

Stars are divisions that have high market share in markets that are growing rapidly. These businesses generate excitement. They also generate a lot of cash due to their high market share. At the same time, they require significant cash to fuel their continued growth in the rapidly expanding market and to fend off competitors who wish to take away their market share. The cash the stars generate usually tends to net out. In that sense, they are similar to dogs, but they continue to have huge upside. Strategic approaches include continuing to fuel the growth and expand market share through market penetration and market development, product development, integration strategies, and even joint ventures. Defensive moves intended to maintain the large market share are also considered. If a star maintains its dominant market share as the market life cycle matures, it moves into the cash cow category; at this point, other competitors drop out and the star requires less cash to fuel the strong financial results. However, if a star fails to maintain its share, it degrades into a dog.

Cash Cows

Cash cows have a dominant market share in markets that are not growing significantly. Because market domination tends to correlate with pricing power, they have significant profit margins. In addition, they require only limited cash investment due to the market's lower growth, meaning they generate significantly more cash than they consume. Strategies for cash cows involve continuing to support the division without having to

EXHIBIT 12.3
BCG Matrix for Company X

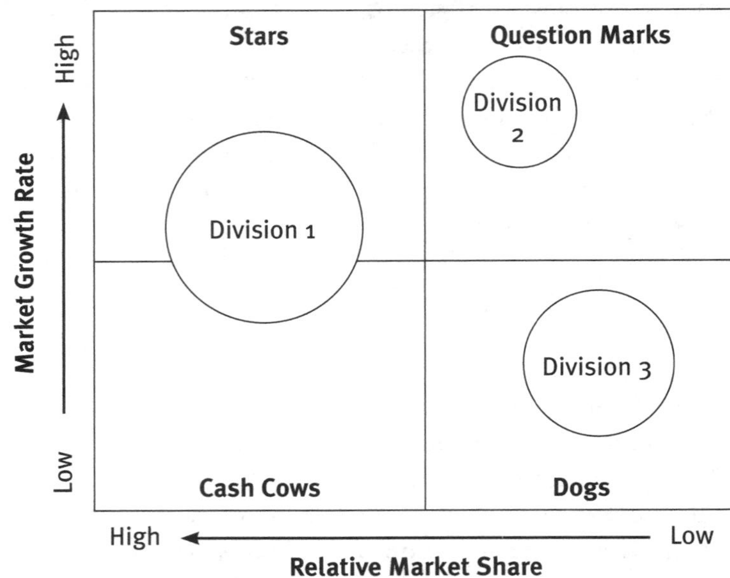

invest significant cash, then using the cash generated to reinvest in turning around dogs or moving question marks into stars.

When divisions are placed on the BCG matrix, they are indicated by a circle. Usually, the size of each circle indicates the relative significance of each business unit to the organization in terms of cash generated (see Exhibit 12.3). Alternatively, the circles could be the same size but with pie slices in each. The pie slice would be shaded to show the relationship between the cash generated by that division (the slice) and the whole.

The BCG matrix allows a quick visualization of a company's portfolio relative to market share, market growth, size of cash contribution, and relative strength or weakness. The matrix can also be used to show a target company and its position relative to its competitors, by placing the company on the matrix and then placing the competitors appropriately. The BCG matrix is the first analysis tool we have seen that begins to suggest strategy in addition to simple analysis.

Reference

Boston Consulting Group (BCG). 1973. "The Experience Curve—Reviewed." Accessed August 17, 2015. www.bcg.com/documents/file13904.pdf.

For your project company, review the previous analyses and develop a BCG matrix. Plot all the divisions or business units of your organization.

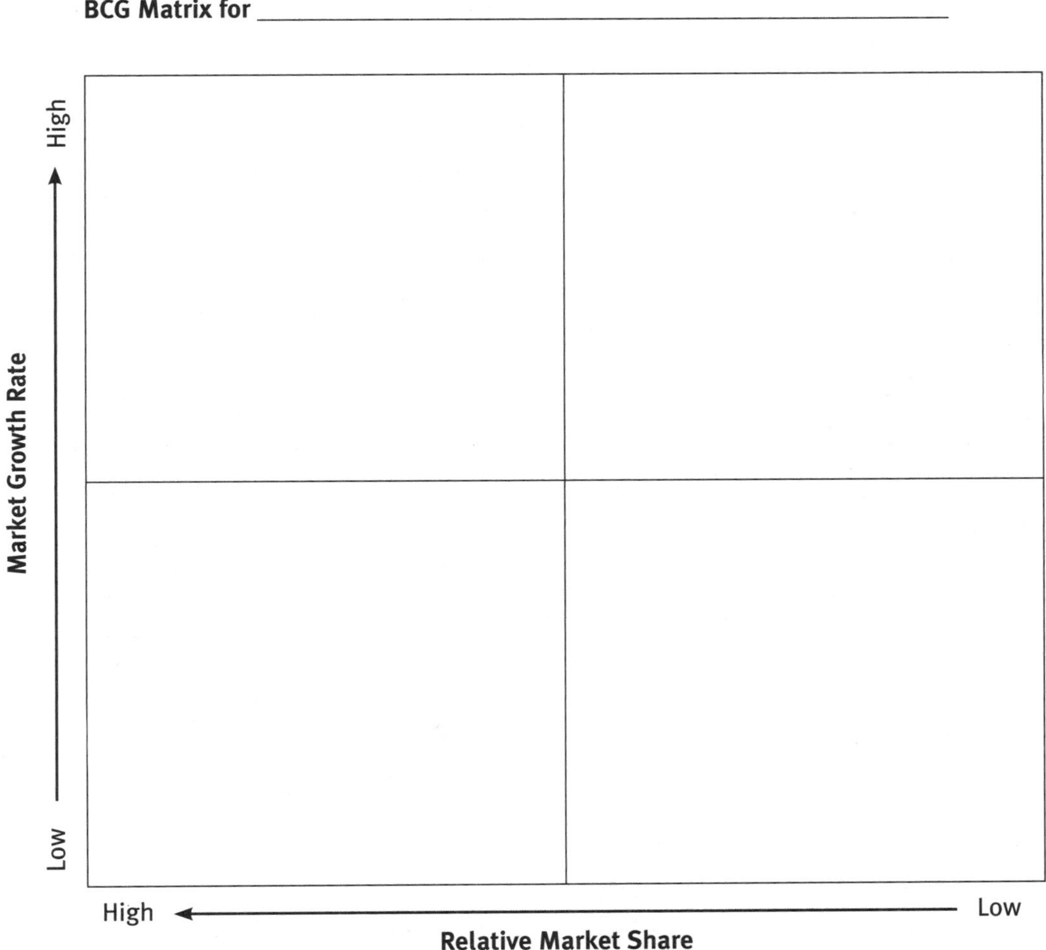

EXERCISE

CHAPTER

13

GENERAL ELECTRIC MATRIX

The General Electric (GE) nine-block business screen, commonly called the GE matrix, was developed by the consulting firm McKinsey & Company. It is similar in many respects to the BCG matrix, but it has surpassed the BCG matrix in popularity. In the GE matrix, the business's overall strength is compared to the overall attractiveness of the market within which the business competes. As in the BCG matrix, multiple divisions can be placed on the GE matrix so that the strategist can quickly take in a great deal of data in a simplified format (see Exhibit 13.1).

The popularity of the GE matrix stems from its flexibility as well as from its ability to include a greater number of variables in the analysis. Whereas the BCG matrix uses the term *market growth* for the vertical axis, the GE matrix uses *market attractiveness*. And where the BCG matrix uses *relative market share* for the horizontal axis, the GE matrix uses *business strength*. Although the differences may seem subtle, the effect on practical application is significant. In the sections ahead, we consider how market attractiveness and business strength are defined.

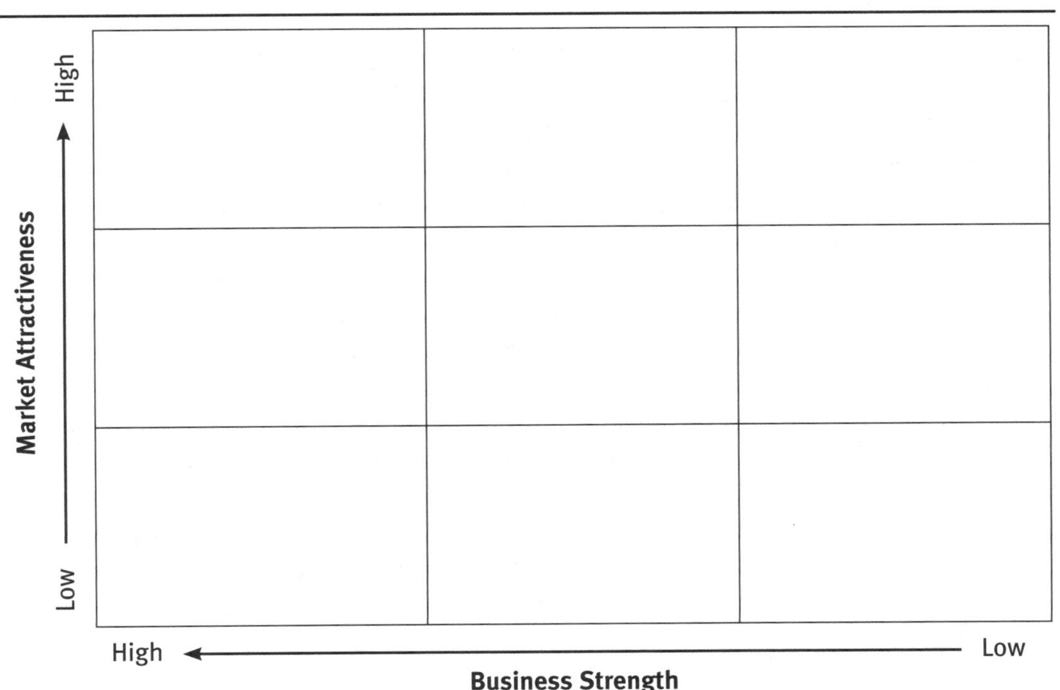

EXHIBIT 13.1
GE Matrix

Market Attractiveness

What makes a market attractive? There is no clear definition. Ultimately, market attractiveness is for the strategist to judge, and as a result, successful strategy development hangs in the balance. One way to define market attractiveness, as with the BCG matrix, is simply to use market growth. But is that a good proxy for how attractive a market is? In reality, market attractiveness is much more complex. The recognition of this complexity is where the GE matrix has an inherent advantage over the BCG matrix. It has the ability to combine an infinite number of variables to arrive at a customized definition of market attractiveness. At the same time, however, this imprecision could also be a drawback.

When determining market attractiveness, the strategist may consider aspects of other industry analysis models, such as Porter's five forces (threat of new entrants, rivalry among existing firms, threat of substitutes, bargaining power of buyers, and bargaining power of sellers) or the opportunities and threats sections of SWOT.

Business Strength

Just as market attractiveness is loosely defined, the same is true for business strength. When considering the strength of a business, the strategist may think of the strengths and weaknesses sections of SWOT. These *SW* issues will likely include market share, as well as such factors as strength of the brand, manufacturing quality, distribution reach, customer loyalty, cost structure, and staff quality.

Constructing the Matrix

When constructing the GE matrix, the analyst first creates a nine-block chart. The vertical axis represents market attractiveness, and the three levels of blocks are labeled "Low," "Medium," and "High" (or, alternatively, "Weak," "Average," and "Strong"). The horizontal axis represents business strength and is divided into the same three levels. The company's divisions are placed on the matrix according to their intersection of market attractiveness and business strength.

When the divisions are placed on the matrix, each is represented by a circle. The size of the circle represents the size of the market within which that particular division competes. Within each division's circle, a pie slice represents that particular division's share within its market. See Exhibit 13.2.

Strategic conclusions can be drawn from each division's position on the GE matrix. Strategies associated with the upper-left corner of the matrix can be loosely described as "grow and build" strategies, and those associated with the lower-right corner can be described as "harvest and divest." "Hold and maintain" strategies are associated with the boxes running from the lower-left corner to the upper-right. More detailed strategic conclusions associated with each of the nine boxes are shown in Exhibit 13.3.

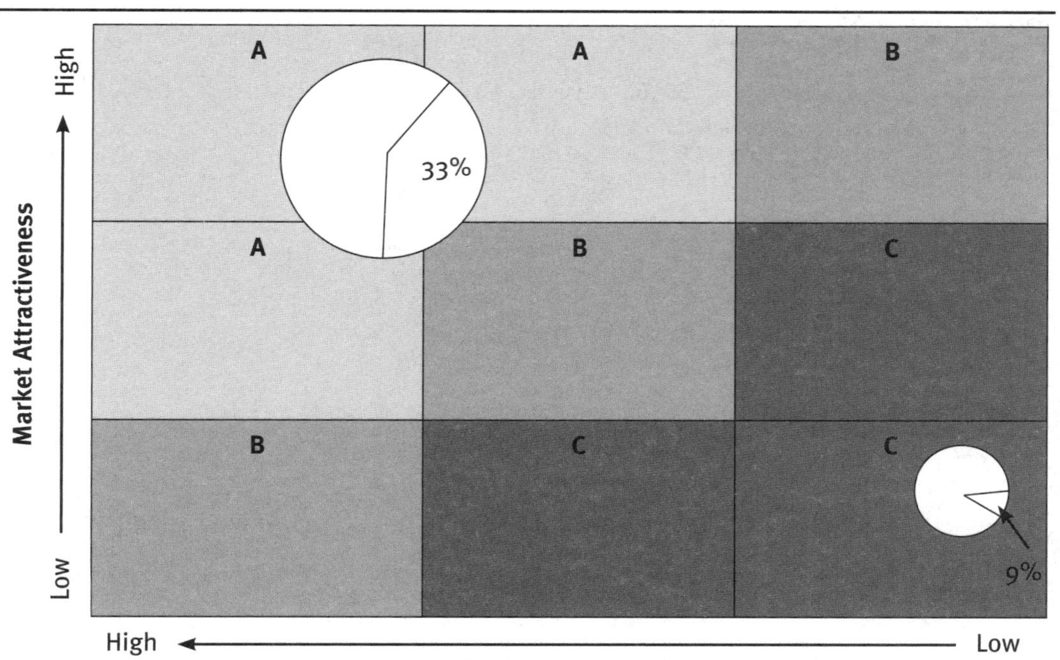

General Strategies on Matrix Location:

(light)	Grow and Build	Integration strategies, intensive strategies
(medium)	Hold and Maintain	Market penetration, product development, joint venture
(dark)	Harvest and Divest	Retrenchment, divestiture, liquidation

EXHIBIT 13.2
GE Matrix with Two Divisions Plotted

EXHIBIT 13.3
Strategic Implications for the GE Matrix

High Attractiveness **Strong Business Strength** The strategy advice for this cell is to invest for growth. Consider the following strategies: Provide maximum investment, diversify, consolidate your position to focus your resources, accept moderate near-term profits to build share.	**High Attractiveness** **Average Business Strength** The strategy advice for this cell is to invest for growth. Consider the following strategies: Build selectively on strength, define the implications of challenging for market leadership, fill weaknesses to avoid vulnerability.	**High Attractiveness** **Weak Business Strength** The strategy advice for this cell is to opportunistically invest for earnings. However, if you can't strengthen your enterprise, you should exit the market. Consider the following strategies: Ride with the market growth, seek niches or specialization, seek an opportunity to increase strength through acquisition.
Medium Attractiveness **Strong Business Strength** The strategy advice for this cell is to selectively invest for growth. Consider the following strategies: Invest heavily in selected segments, establish a ceiling for the market share you wish to achieve, seek attractive new segments to apply strengths.	**Medium Attractiveness** **Average Business Strength** The strategy advice for this cell is to selectively invest for earnings. Consider the following strategies: Segment the market to find a more attractive position, make contingency plans to protect your vulnerable position.	**Medium Attractiveness** **Weak Business Strength** The strategy advice for this cell is to preserve for harvest. Consider the following strategies: Act to preserve or boost cash flow as you exit the business, seek an opportunistic sale, seek a way to increase your strengths.
Low Attractiveness **Strong Business Strength** The strategy advice for this cell is to selectively invest for earnings. Consider the following strategies: Defend strengths, shift resources to attractive segments, examine ways to revitalize the industry, time your exit by monitoring for harvest or divestment timing.	**Low Attractiveness** **Average Business Strength** The strategy advice for this cell is to restructure, harvest, or divest. Consider the following strategies: Make only essential commitments, prepare to divest, shift resources to a more attractive segment.	**Low Attractiveness** **Weak Business Strength** The strategy advice for this cell is to harvest or divest. You should exit the market or prune the product line.

Source: Business Resource Software, Inc. (2015).

Reference

Business Resource Software, Inc. 2015. "Analysis of Your Enterprise Position." Accessed June 23. www.brs-inc.com/models/model17.asp.

For your project organization, review the previous analyses and develop a GE matrix in the space provided.

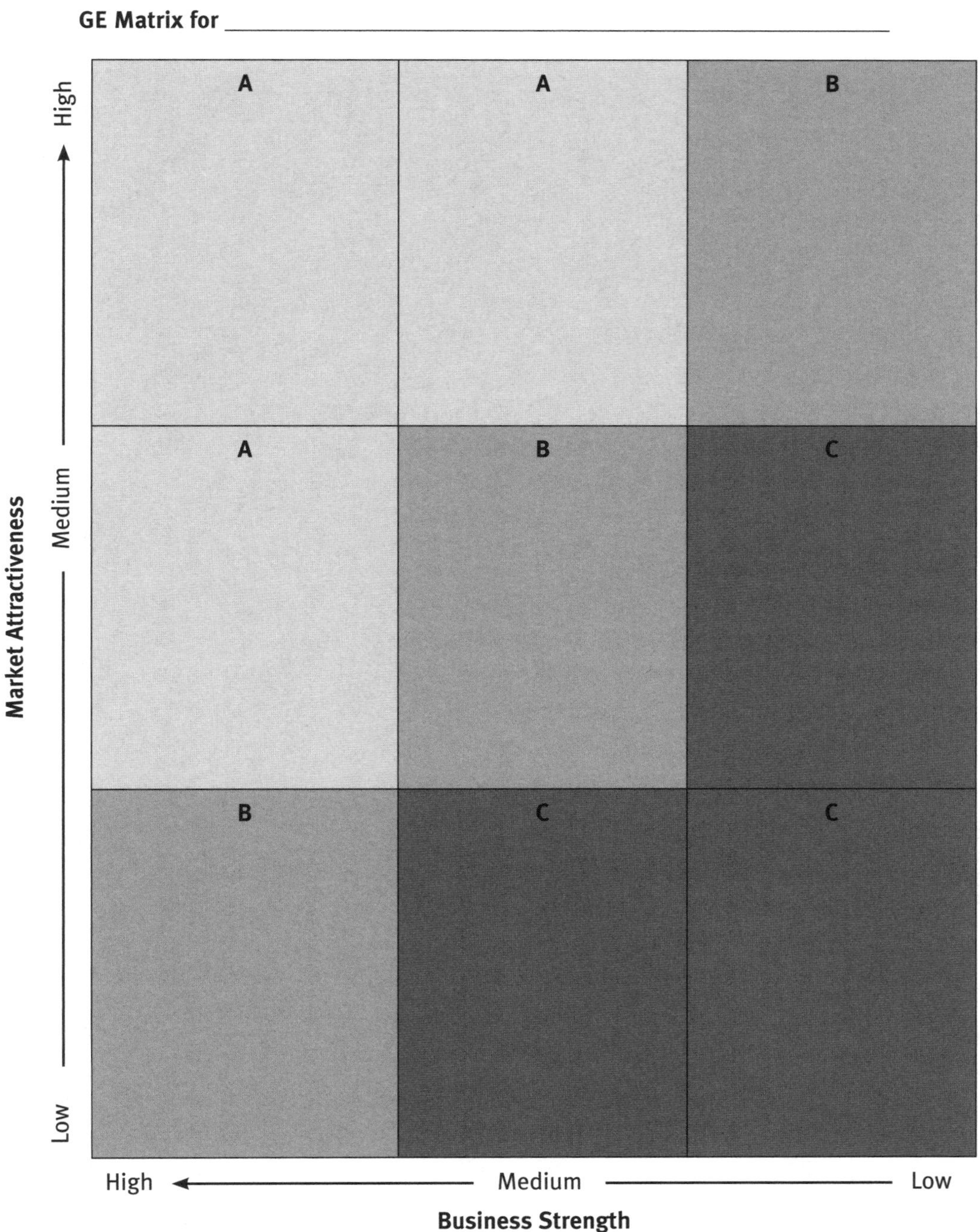

CHAPTER

14

McKINSEY 7S MODEL

Developed by the McKinsey management consulting group in the late 1970s, the 7S framework changed the way people thought about organizational effectiveness. "A previous focus of managers was on organization as structure—who does what, who reports to whom, and the like. As organizations grew in size and complexity, the more critical question became one of coordination" (McKinsey & Company 2008).

The 7S model takes its name from seven components: strategy, structure, systems, staff, skills, style, and shared values (see Exhibit 14.1). The sections that follow provide questions to ask and issues to consider when assessing each of these elements.

Strategy

When you analyze strategy, ask yourself how well your organization's current strategy has enabled it to reach its goals. Areas to consider may include the following (Braintree Group 2015):

- Marketing strategy
- Distribution
- Product or service development

EXHIBIT 14.1
McKinsey 7S Model

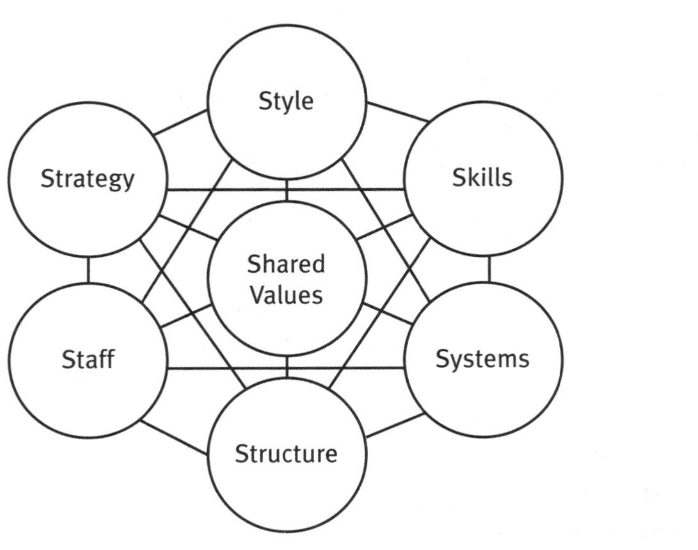

Source: McKinsey & Company (2008).

- Business development
- Customer service
- Understanding of external market factors

Structure

Organizational structure—the second *S*—determines how well an organization can respond to new challenges and customer requirements. Companies with flat structures tend to allow more autonomy for individual business units and managers, enabling them to respond quickly to changing market conditions. More traditional, hierarchical organizations tend to be less responsive. However, they tend to have greater central management control and are better able to leverage the buying and selling power of the whole business (Braintree Group 2015).

Systems

The third *S* involves the organization's managerial processes, systems, and business tools. Ask yourself: Do these elements allow the organization to run efficiently and deliver good customer service, or do they hinder the pursuit of these goals? Areas to consider include the following (Braintree Group 2015):

- Customer service, research and development (R&D), sales, and marketing operations
- Collection of management information
- Financial management
- Information technology
- Internal communications

Staff

Organizations depend heavily on their staffs. This point is especially true in healthcare, where poor staff interactions can ruin a customer's relationship with an organization. The ability of an organization to recruit, train, and retain a skilled and talented staff is particularly important (Braintree Group 2015).

Skills

The skills of an organization determine its ability to

- provide innovative products and services,
- differentiate itself from its competitors,
- charge premium prices, and
- defend and grow market share.

Highly skilled organizations tend to invest in equipment, R&D, and staff recruitment and development. They tend to have a strong understanding of their markets, reward success, and maintain a no-blame culture (Braintree Group 2015).

Style

The style with which managers approach the business tends to be reflected throughout the organization. Managers who provide a supportive and enabling approach to staff, for instance, will often find that the same positive approach is passed along to customers (Braintree Group 2015). Style may also be thought of as "culture." Healthcare managers and administrators work with as diverse a group of employees as one could imagine. All ages, genders, ethnic backgrounds, shapes, and sizes can be found in healthcare organizations. Therefore, we must understand how to work with a broad intersection of people from all walks of life. We must lead effectively with a style that can transcend inherent differences and make the organization function as a cohesive unit.

Shared Values

The final *S* is shared values. To be truly successful, the entire organization needs to work toward the same goals and values. Effective internal communications are key to ensuring that staff members are aware of the goals and values and, further, that they understand why those goals and values are so important.

Applying the 7S Model

In keeping with the 7S model's emphasis on coordination, you should apply the framework with the following key points in mind (JISC InfoNet 2008):

- Focus on the links between each of the *S*s rather on the *S*s themselves. The links are key to identifying the organization's strengths and weaknesses. No *S* is a strength or a weakness in its own right; only its degree of support (or lack thereof) for the other *S*s is relevant.
- The model highlights how a change made in any one *S* will have an impact on all the others. Thus, for a planned change to be effective, changes in one *S* should be accompanied by complementary changes in the others.

For more information, you can watch a short video from McKinsey & Company on the 7S framework: www.mckinseyquarterly.com/Enduring_ideas_The_7-S_Framework_2123?pagenum=1#interactive_7s.

References

Braintree Group. 2015. "McKinsey's 7 S's Capability Audit." Accessed June 25. www.braintreegroup.co.uk/mckinseys-7-ss/4584486892.

JISC InfoNet. 2008. "7S Model." Published April 6. www.jiscinfonet.ac.uk/tools/seven-s-model/.

McKinsey & Company. 2008. "Enduring Ideas: The 7-S Framework." *McKinsey Quarterly*. Published March. www.mckinseyquarterly.com/Enduring_ideas_The_7-S_Framework_2123.

CHAPTER

15

LIFE CYCLE ANALYSIS

Life cycle analysis assesses products, companies, or industries by analyzing the current stage in their life cycle. Although numerous life cycle models exist, researchers have generally identified five main phases in a life cycle:

- Birth
- Growth
- Maturity
- Revival
- Decline

Exhibit 15.1 illustrates a company's path through the five phases. As a successful company ages, it tends to grow both in size and in administrative complexity. As a company declines, its size and complexity contract. As a company moves through the life cycle, each phase has certain attributes that are commonly observed relative to the company's "situation," "organization," and "innovation and strategy." Miller and Friesen (1984) aggregated data from past studies and created the chart shown in Exhibit 15.2.

Birth Phase Strategy

According to Miller and Friesen (1984, 1169–70), organizations in the birth stage are "attempting to establish for the first time a viable product-market strategy. This is achieved

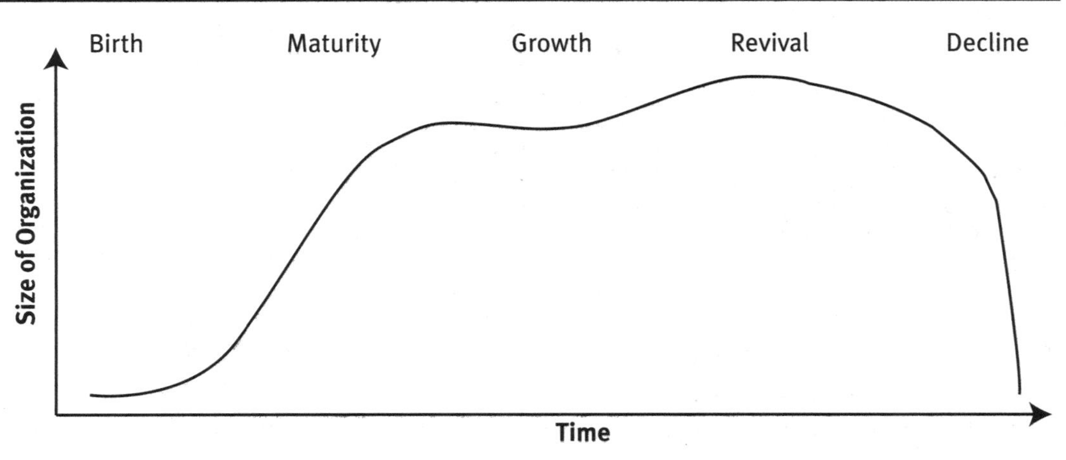

EXHIBIT 15.1
Life Cycle Analysis

EXHIBIT 15.2
Life Cycle Phases and Attributes

Corporate Life Cycle

Phase	Situation	Organization	Innovation & Strategy
Birth Phase:	Small firm Young Dominated by owner/ manager Homogeneous/placid environment	Informal structure Undifferentiated Power highly centralized Crude information-processing & decision-making methods	Considerable innovation in product lines Niche strategy Substantial risk taking
Growth Phase:	Medium sized Older Multiple shareholders A more heterogeneous & competitive environment	Some formalization of structure Functional basis of organization Moderate differentiation Somewhat less centralized Initial development of formal information-processing & decision-making tools	Broadening of product-market scope into closely related areas Incremental innovation in product lines Rapid growth
Maturity Phase:	Larger Even older Dispersed ownership Heterogeneous & competitive environment	Formal, bureaucratic structure Functional basis of organization Moderate differentiation Moderate centralization Information processing & decision making same as growth stage	Consolidation of product-market strategy Focus on efficiently supplying a well-defined market Conservatism Slow growth
Revival Phase:	Very large Very heterogeneous, competitive, dynamic	Divisional basis of organization High differentiation Sophisticated control, scanning, and communications in information processing; more formal analysis in decision making	Strategy of product-market diversification; movement into some unrelated markets High level of risk taking & planning Substantial innovation Rapid growth
Decline Phase:	Market size Homogeneous and competitive environment	Formal, bureaucratic structure Mostly functional basis of organization Moderate differentiations and centralization Less sophisticated information-processing systems and decision-making methods	Low level of innovation Price cutting Consolidation of product market Liquidation of subsidiaries Risk aversion & conservatism

Source: Reprinted with permission from Miller and Friesen (1984).

mainly by trial and error as efforts are made to change products and services in a manner that generates distinctive competences. This generally involves major and frequent product or service innovations and the conscious pursuit of a niche strategy." Because companies in the birth phase are small and have no established reputation, they do not directly confront their more powerful competitors. Instead, they find gaps, or niches, in the market that are not being filled, and they fill and defend these niches by making innovations. Miller and Friesen observed "a tendency for firms in the birth phase to use middlemen in marketing mainly to achieve economies of distribution. Firms were simply not substantial enough to set up their own channels of distribution."

We can see this approach in smaller health-related businesses, including some contemporary drug stores: Small operations are opening and using niche strategy to get off the ground initially, and then, if successful, they begin to move on to the next phase.

Growth Phase Strategy

Miller and Friesen (1984, 1170–71) identify the emphasis of the second stage as growth and early diversification: "Product lines are broadened. But this generally results in a more complete array of products for a given market rather than positions in widely varying markets. Efforts are also devoted to incrementally tailoring products to new markets, while less stress is placed on major or dramatic product innovations. Market segmentation begins to play a role, with managers trying to identify specific subgroups of customers and to make small product or service modifications in order to better serve them. In other words, the niche strategy is often abandoned as broader markets are addressed." Organizations in the growth phase are bigger and stronger than those in the birth phase, and they are better able to lobby with various levels of government. They may also acquire subsidiaries in their efforts to diversify. An acquisition of this nature, Miller and Friesen write, "generally takes the form of buying out much smaller competing enterprises in the same industry rather than diversifying into new industries. The acquired firms are usually integrated into the functionally-based structure rather than left as independent divisions." Growth phase strategies can be seen in various healthcare sectors, especially as systemization takes place across the United States.

Maturity Phase Strategy

Firms in the maturity phase are conservative, according to Miller and Friesen (1984, 1171–72): "They do not perform many major innovations, engage in very few efforts at diversification or acquisition, and fail even to make many incremental changes to the products or services being offered. Indeed, the tendency, more than in any other phase, is to follow the competition; to wait for competitors to lead the way in innovating and, then, to imitate the innovations if they prove to be necessary." Markets in the maturity phase are slightly broader than in the growth phase, and fewer firms opt for a niche strategy. Firms try to arrange for a stable, negotiated environment by fixing prices and lobbying with the government. "The goal appears to be to improve the efficiency and profitability of operations. This is achieved by avoiding costly changes in product lines, ensuring favorable prices via collusion, and lobbying for barriers to foreign competition. A stable and circumscribed product line is sold in traditional markets, the emphasis being upon economical production and the preservation of sales volume."

Revival Phase Strategy

Many life cycle models do not show a revival stage; instead, they simply show maturity leading to decline. Real-world observation shows that some companies do in fact move from maturity to decline, but many others experience a "post-maturity" revival stage prior to decline.

According to Miller and Friesen (1984, 1173–74), "The revival phase is in many ways the most exciting of the five. Remarkable changes begin to take place in the product-market strategies being followed. For example, there are more major and minor product-line and service innovations than in any other period. Also, new markets are entered for the first time as firms become more diversified." This diversification sometimes involves the acquisition of firms in different industries. Market segmentation further defines discrete parts of the environment, and firms differentiate product lines accordingly. Miller and Friesen continue: "Essentially, firms experience dramatic diversification in their products and markets. Their growth does not simply result in an increase in size but an expansion of product-market scope. There is a movement from one market to many, reversing the stagnation of the maturity phase." Because of their size, market power, visibility, and occasional acquisitions, some firms in the revival phase lobby with the government to avoid interference with expansion, to obtain protection against imports, and to avoid antitrust lawsuits.

Decline Phase Strategy

Firms in the decline stage react to adversity in their markets by becoming stagnant, according to Miller and Friesen (1984, 1174–75). "They try to conserve resources depleted by poor performance by abstaining from product or service innovation. Product lines are rendered antiquated so that it becomes necessary to cut prices to maintain sales. Firms seem to be caught in something of a vicious circle. Their sales are poor because their product lines are unappealing. This reduces profits and makes for scarcer financial resources, which in turn cause any significant product line changes to seem too expensive." As a result, changes are avoided, and product lines become even more outdated. "It's almost as though no particular strategy were being pursued; the firms just muddle through."

Exhibit 15.3 displays survey results concerning the reasons that companies decline. Note that only 8 percent of the companies surveyed attributed their decline to lack of sales or revenue. The rest of the reasons are management decisions or attributes.

EXHIBIT 15.3 Reasons for Company Decline

Reasons for Decline	
Too much debt	28%
Inadequate leadership	17%
Poor planning	14%
Failure to change	11%
Inexperienced management	9%
Not enough revenue	8%

Source: *Businessweek* (2003).

EXHIBIT 15.4 Critical Problems Matrix

	Early Stage	Late Stage
Little or No Competition	1. Lack of dependencies and constraints in pursuing goals Critical problems: (a) Resources (b) Marketing approach (c) Formalization of structure	2. Environment neither threatening nor constraining Critical problems: (a) Stabilizing firm's position (b) Formalization & control (c) Stability
Intense Competition	3. Turbulent environment—may constrain or dictate actions Critical problems: (a) Identify niches (b) Monitor competition (c) Realignment of the firm vis-à-vis the competition	4. Muddling behavior, simply reacting Critical problems: (a) Maintain market position (b) Further image via focus & differentiation strategies (c) Cost control

Source: Reprinted with permission from Dodge, Fullerton, and Robbins (1994).

Life Cycle / Competition Matrix

Dodge, Fullerton, and Robbins (1994) suggest a different way to consider the organizational life cycle. First, they group organizations into either early stages of development or late stages of development. They then consider the level of competition the organizations are experiencing. The resulting four-block matrix displays common critical problems faced by companies in each block (see Exhibit 15.4). Strategies can be developed to address the critical problems. Exhibit 15.5 demonstrates this approach using the example of Toyota Motor Corporation and its competitors.

EXHIBIT 15.5 Toyota Life Cycle

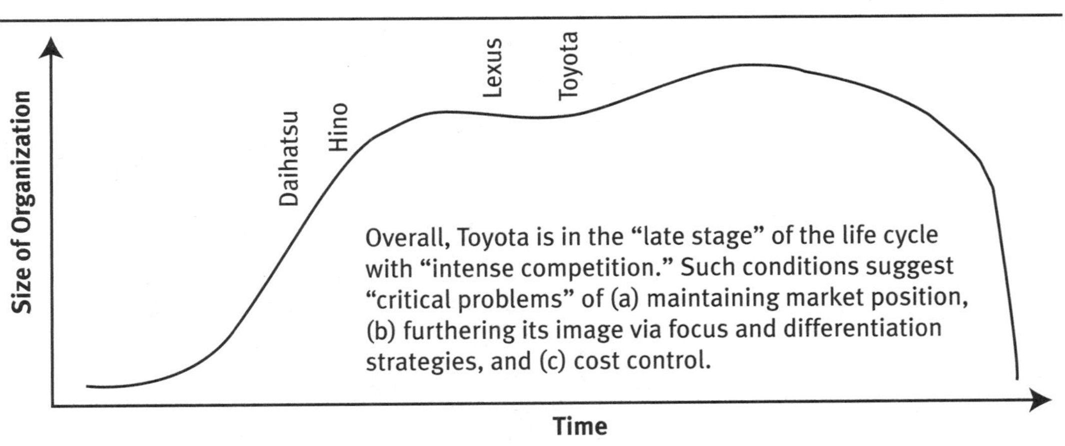

Daihatsu Motor Co., Ltd., produces mini cars and compact cars primarily for the Japanese market. The car market in Japan is mature. Exports are a growth opportunity and represent 30 percent of sales. Contracted engine production is another growth opportunity.

Hino Motors, Ltd., manufactures and sells trucks and buses, light-commercial vehicles, passenger vehicles (commissioned from Toyota Motor Corporation), and various types of engines and spare parts. It is based in Japan and sells worldwide. The market is mature, but Hino continues to grow through international expansion.

Lexus manufactures passenger vehicles for the North American market. This market is mature and competitive.

Toyota manufactures passenger vehicles for the worldwide market. Certain segments are mature (North America, Western Europe), and other markets represent growth opportunities (developing countries). Unit sales have consistently increased year after year.

References

Businessweek. 2003. "The Keys to Failure." *Businessweek* August 25, 14.

Dodge, H. R., S. Fullerton, and J. E. Robbins. 1994. "Stage of the Organizational Life Cycle and Competition as Mediators of Problem Perception for Small Businesses." *Strategic Management Journal* 15 (2): 121–34.

Miller, D., and P. Friesen. 1984. "A Longitudinal Study of the Corporate Life Cycle." *Management Science* 30 (10): 1161–83.

In the space provided, develop a life cycle analysis—with explanations and implications for strategy—for your project organization.

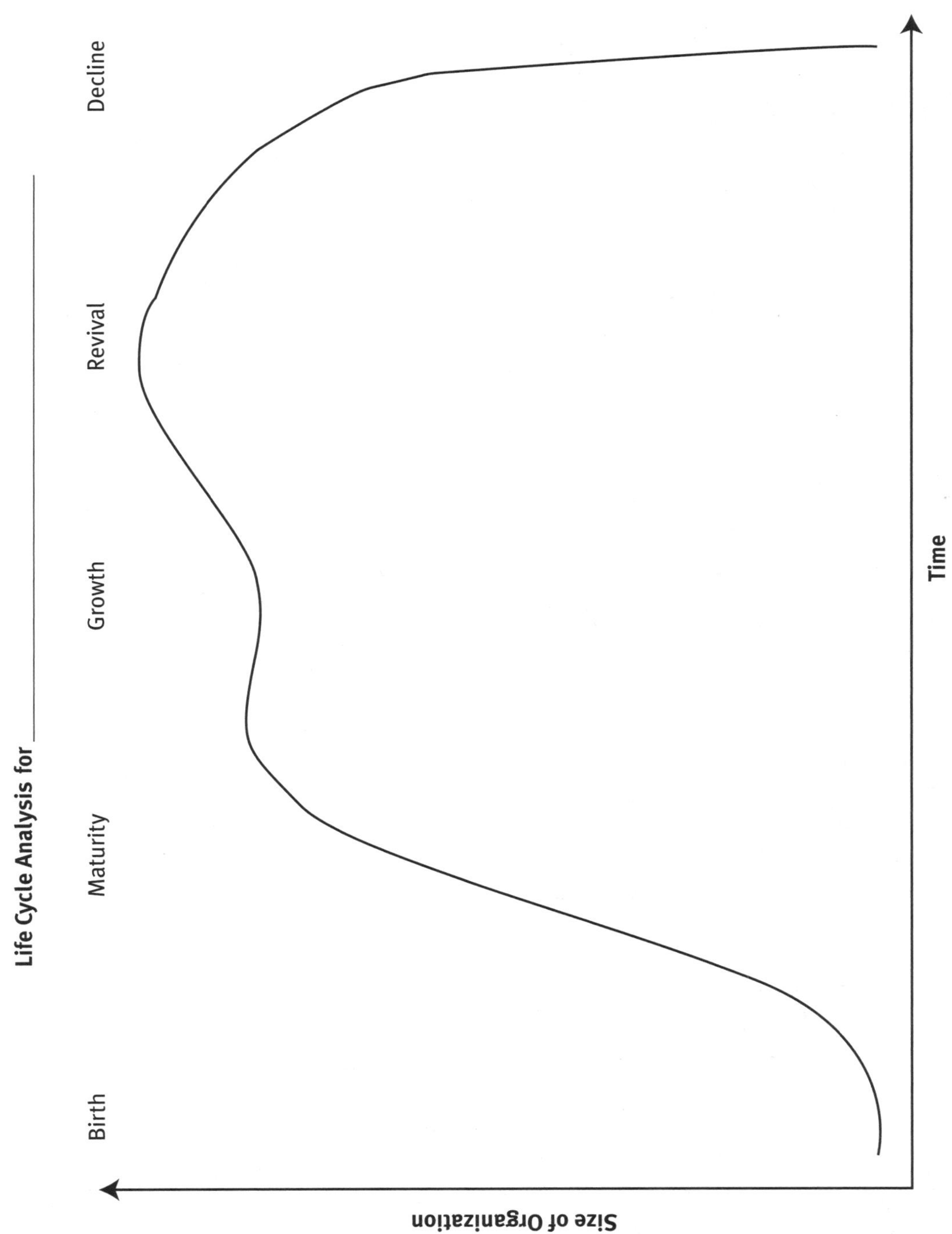

EXERCISE

EXERCISE

Explanation:

-
-
-
-
-
-
-

Implications for Strategy from Life Cycle Analysis:

1.
2.
3.
4.
5.
6.
7.
8.
9.
10.

CHAPTER

16

ORGANIZATIONAL CULTURE ANALYSIS

Organizational culture can be defined as the system of shared values, meanings, and beliefs held by organizational members that determines, to a large degree, how the members act toward one another (Robbins and Coulter 2009). It is often referred to as "how we do things around here." A strong, positive culture can improve organizational performance, whereas a weak or negative culture can detract from organizational performance. To say that values are shared implies that they are passed between existing employees and are passed on to new employees.

Consider how Starbucks brings a new barista into the company. After a person who "fits" the Starbucks culture has been selected, the new employee is put through weeks of introductory training, followed by on-the-job instruction and mentorship. The key to this onboarding process is the transmission of "how we do things around here." The Starbucks values, motives, and meanings are indoctrinated so that a barista is a barista whether you go to a Starbucks in Gary, Indiana, or in New York City. The same is true for Chick-Fil-A, which is known for its thorough screening and training and its emphasis on organizational values. Its onboarding processes stand in contrast to those of most fast-food competitors. Similarly, stark differences can be seen when comparing the slow-moving, bureaucratic culture of domestic automotive companies to the empowering and innovative culture of a company like Google.

In healthcare, culture plays a significant role in the success of the organization, and it comprises many factors. Culture, as defined by Longest and Darr (2014), includes the organization's values and ethics, its cohesiveness, its philosophy about continuous quality improvement, its customers and employees, and the compatibility of culture with the mission. The difficulty is putting your finger on the pulse of culture. If you are inside the organization, you will have a strong opportunity to identify the cultural aspects. If you are on the outside, you will need to "read the tea leaves" by analyzing what is said in annual reports, by Wall Street analysts, and in articles written about the organization.

What do the coffee and fast-food industries have to do with healthcare? Not much, usually, unless the products they serve cause some harm to the customer. But culture plays an extremely important role in healthcare organizations, and the examples of these successful organizations provide a great start to understanding how it works. Having the right people on board, and in the right seats, is essential if the organization is to reach its full potential.

Another key to organizational success in contemporary healthcare is cultural competency. We see a diverse patient population, and we must be able to serve the needs of everyone. According to the Substance Abuse and Mental Health Services Administration (2015), cultural competency is a set of congruent behaviors, attitudes, and policies that come together in a system, through an agency, or among professionals and enable that system, that agency, or those professionals to work effectively in cross-cultural situations. A report by the Lewin Group (2002) identified seven performance areas that practitioners can use to assess an organization's level of cultural competence:

- Organizational values—the perspective, attitudes, and commitment concerning the worth and importance of cultural competence
- Governance—the use of goal setting, policy making, and other methods of oversight to help ensure culturally competent care
- Planning and monitoring/evaluation—the mechanisms, processes, and systems in place to assess cultural competence and to guide cultural competence planning
- Communication—the exchange of information between the organization and the population, and between members of the staff, in ways that promote cultural competence
- Staff development—the efforts to ensure that staff and other service providers have the attitudes, knowledge, and skills necessary for culturally competent care
- Organizational infrastructure—the organizational resources needed to deliver or facilitate the delivery of culturally competent services
- Services/interventions—the extent to which the organization delivers services in a culturally competent manner

References

Lewin Group. 2002. "Indicators of Cultural Competence in Health Care Delivery Organizations: An Organizational Cultural Competence Assessment Profile." Published April. www.hrsa.gov/culturalcompetence/healthdlvr.pdf.

Longest, B. B., and K. Darr. 2014. *Managing Health Services Organizations and Systems*, 6th ed. Baltimore, MD: Health Professions Press.

Robbins, S. P., and M. K. Coulter. 2009. *Management*, 10th ed. Upper Saddle River, NJ: Prentice Hall.

Substance Abuse and Mental Health Services Administration. 2015. "Ensuring Cultural Competence at the Organizational Level." Accessed March 30. https://captus.samhsa.gov/access-resources/ensuring-cultural-competence-organizational-level.

To the extent that you can for your project company, identify dimensions such as the following and use them to describe the organizational culture.

Dimensions of Organizational Culture (Robbins and Coulter 2009)
Attention to detail—the degree to which employees are expected to show precision, analysis, and attention to detail
Outcome orientation—the extent to which managers focus on results and outcomes regardless of how they are achieved
People orientation—the degree to which management takes into account the effects of its decisions on the people in the organization
Team orientation—the extent to which work is organized around teams rather than individuals
Aggressiveness—the degree to which employees are aggressive and competitive rather than cooperative
Stability—the extent to which organizational decisions and actions emphasize maintaining the status quo
Innovation and risk taking—the degree to which employees are encouraged to be innovative and take risks

EXERCISE

Does the organizational culture hold the company back, or does the culture spur innovation?

Does the culture support the company status quo, or does the culture need to change to support new strategies you are developing? If the culture needs to change, you need to develop a specific strategy to change it.

CHAPTER

17

SWOT: INTERNAL STRENGTHS AND WEAKNESSES

As we discussed in Chapter 9, SWOT analysis looks at a company's strengths, weaknesses, opportunities, and threats. It brings together information from various analyses to help form a cohesive assessment of the company. SWOT does not identify particular strategies, but it identifies issues that may need to be strategically addressed. The SWOT analysis is split into two dimensions: internal issues and external issues (see Exhibit 17.1). In Chapter 9, we examined the external factors—opportunities and threats (*OT*). In this chapter, we will look at the internal strengths and weaknesses (*SW*).

A strength can be thought of as any internal attribute of the organization that is helpful in achieving corporate objectives. Strengths have positive impacts on your company's profitability and competitive well-being. Positive impacts could involve such conditions as strong cash position, effective corporate culture, or superior manufacturing capability.

A weakness can be thought of as any internal attribute of the organization that is a hindrance in achieving corporate objectives. Weaknesses pose obstacles to your company's profitability and competitive well-being. Such obstacles could be in the same categories as the issues mentioned above—for instance, poor cash position, weak corporate culture, or inferior manufacturing capability.

To begin the *SW* portion of your SWOT, first focus on the internal factors that, either now or in the future, could impact your company. Consider the critical success factors that pertain to your company's environment. This information should draw upon your research about the organization in particular, as well as the industry and external environment in general.

You have previously assessed these issues to develop your financial ratio analysis, BCG matrix, GE matrix, McKinsey 7S analysis, life cycle analysis, and organizational culture analysis. Your Porter's five forces analysis, PEST analysis, and competitive benchmark analysis may provide additional clues. A publicly traded company's Securities and Exchange Commission filings—such as the annual report, 10-K, and 10-Q—can also

EXHIBIT 17.1
Dimensions of SWOT Analysis

Internal:	Strengths	Weaknesses
External:	Opportunities	Threats

EXHIBIT 17.2
Strength and Weakness Analysis Example

Strengths
1. Local market dominance
2. Caring staff
3. Excellent administration
4. Good location
5. Outstanding facilities
6. Strong community support
7. Excellent board of trustees
8. Expanding to meet growth
9. Center of regional healthcare
10. Technology

Weaknesses
1. Weak process to manage low-income population
2. Inability to manage population without health coverage
3. No process to address transient market
4. Difficulty recruiting providers
5. Reputation of the facility
6. Not addressing changes in reimbursement
7. Staff turnover
8. Nursing shortage
9. Need for technical staff
10. Limited resources in mental health

provide a wealth of information for the SWOT analysis. Review all those analyses and identify the issues that could become a competitive threat or could create a competitive opportunity for your company.

Typically, you should identify about ten strengths and ten weaknesses. Note again that you are not proposing strategies or solutions here. You are identifying critical issues that will need to be addressed in subsequent strategy development sections. Exhibit 17.2 provides a sample analysis using the hypothetical example that was introduced in Chapter 9.

EXERCISE

For your project company, review the previous analyses, consider the critical success factors in the firm's industry, and develop the SW portion of SWOT. What are the implications for strategy?

SW(OT) Analysis of ______________________________

Internal:	**Strengths**	**Weaknesses**
	1.	1.
	2.	2.
	3.	3.
	4.	4.
	5.	5.
	6.	6.
	7.	7.
	8.	8.
	9.	9.
	10.	10.

E X E R C I S E

Implications for Strategy:

1.

2.

3.

4.

5.

6.

7.

8.

9.

10.

CHAPTER

18

INTERNAL FACTOR EVALUATION

Just as an external factor evaluation (EFE) organizes and evaluates the *OT* section of SWOT (see discussion in Chapter 10), an internal factor evaluation (IFE) addresses the *SW* section—the internal strengths and weaknesses. The IFE produces a numeric score that reflects the gravity of each issue listed. The score will correspond to certain standard strategies that will be discussed in Chapter 19.

As you did with the EFE analysis, note that not every item you identified in the *SW* section of your SWOT analysis is of equal strength or equal weakness. Some distinction needs to be made between the "great" strengths and weaknesses and the "could be" strengths and weaknesses. To make these distinctions, review the sample list from the previous chapter, repeated in Exhibit 18.1.

The strategist evaluates each strength and weakness and applies a weighting system. The total when all of the weights have been applied and added is exactly 1.00.

EXHIBIT 18.1 Internal Strengths and Weaknesses

Strengths
1. Local market dominance
2. Caring staff
3. Excellent administration
4. Good location
5. Outstanding facilities
6. Strong community support
7. Excellent board of trustees
8. Expanding to meet growth
9. Center of regional healthcare
10. Technology

Weaknesses
1. Weak process to manage low-income population
2. Inability to manage population without health coverage
3. No process to address transient market
4. Difficulty recruiting providers
5. Reputation of the facility
6. Not addressing changes in reimbursement
7. Staff turnover
8. Nursing shortage
9. Need for technical staff
10. Limited resources in mental health

EXHIBIT 18.2 Weighting of Strengths and Weaknesses

Start of IFE Analysis

Strengths	Weight
1. Local market dominance	0.100
2. Caring staff	0.050
3. Excellent administration	0.050
4. Good location	0.025
5. Outstanding facilities	0.050
6. Strong community support	0.025
7. Excellent board of trustees	0.025
8. Expanding to meet growth	0.050
9. Center of regional healthcare	0.050
10. Technology	0.075

Weaknesses	Weight
1. Weak process to manage low-income population	0.050
2. Inability to manage population without health coverage	0.100
3. No process to address transient market	0.025
4. Difficulty recruiting providers	0.025
5. Reputation of the facility	0.050
6. Not addressing changes in reimbursement	0.100
7. Staff turnover	0.050
8. Nursing shortage	0.025
9. Need for technical staff	0.025
10. Limited resources in mental health	0.050
Total weight:	1.00

Each individual factor, therefore, receives some portion of 1.00. The size of that portion reflects the strategist's subjective evaluation of how important each internal factor is to successful competition within the firm's industry. The more important the factor, the higher is the weight assigned. Building on the previous example, Exhibit 18.2 shows the weights assigned to the individual strengths and weaknesses. The total of 1.00 is the sum of the whole column, including both strengths and weaknesses.

The table shows, for instance, that the weakness associated with managing a significant population without health coverage is deemed to be more significant than the strength of the organization's technology, administration, or facilities. Note that there is no one "correct" weight for any factor. The accuracy of the analysis depends on the strategist; careful research and a clear understanding of the company and industry are essential.

Once weights have been assigned to the importance of each factor in the industry, the strategist now focuses on how significant each strength or weakness is for the company. Strengths and weaknesses are rated on a scale of 3–4 for strengths and 1–2 for weaknesses, as shown here:

4 = major strength
3 = minor strength
1 = major weakness
2 = minor weakness

The rating for each factor is once again subjective on the part of the strategist and should be based on research. These ratings are not added up, so there are no constraints on how the numbers may be distributed. Once the ratings have been applied, each factor's rating is multiplied by its weight to yield a weighted score for the factor. Exhibit 18.3 continues this chapter's example.

The IFE analysis yields a total score when the column of individual scores is summed. This score can be used in an internal–external (I/E) matrix, which corresponds to a standard table of strategic responses. We will explore these steps in the next chapter.

EXHIBIT 18.3
IFE Total Score

IFE Analysis

Strengths	Weight*	Rating†	Score
1. Local market dominance	0.100	4	0.4
2. Caring staff	0.050	3	0.15
3. Excellent administration	0.050	4	0.2
4. Good location	0.025	4	0.1
5. Outstanding facilities	0.050	3	0.15
6. Strong community support	0.025	4	0.1
7. Excellent board of trustees	0.025	3	0.075
8. Expanding to meet growth	0.050	4	0.2
9. Center of regional healthcare	0.050	3	0.15
10. Technology	0.075	4	0.3

Weaknesses	Weight	Rating	Score
1. Weak process to manage low-income population	0.050	1	0.05
2. Inability to manage population without health coverage	0.100	1	0.1
3. No process to address transient market	0.025	2	0.05
4. Difficulty recruiting providers	0.025	1	0.025
5. Reputation of the facility	0.050	2	0.1
6. Not addressing changes in reimbursement	0.100	1	0.1
7. Staff turnover	0.050	1	0.05
8. Nursing shortage	0.025	1	0.025
9. Need for technical staff	0.025	1	0.025
10. Limited resources in mental health	0.050	1	0.05
Total weight:	1.00	**Total score:**	2.400

* Weight is industry specific.
† Rating is organization specific.

EXERCISE

For your project organization, review the previous analyses and develop an IFE analysis.

IFE Analysis of ______________________________

Strengths	Weight	Rating	Score
1.			
2.			
3.			
4.			
5.			
6.			
7.			
8.			
9.			
10.			

Rating scale:
4 = major strength
3 = minor strength

(continued)

EXERCISE

Weaknesses	Weight	Rating	Score
1.			
2.			
3.			
4.			
5.			
6.			
7.			
8.			
9.			
10.			

Rating scale:
1 = major weakness
2 = minor weakness

Total weight: ☐ **Score:** ☐

PART

IV

INTEGRATIVE ANALYSIS

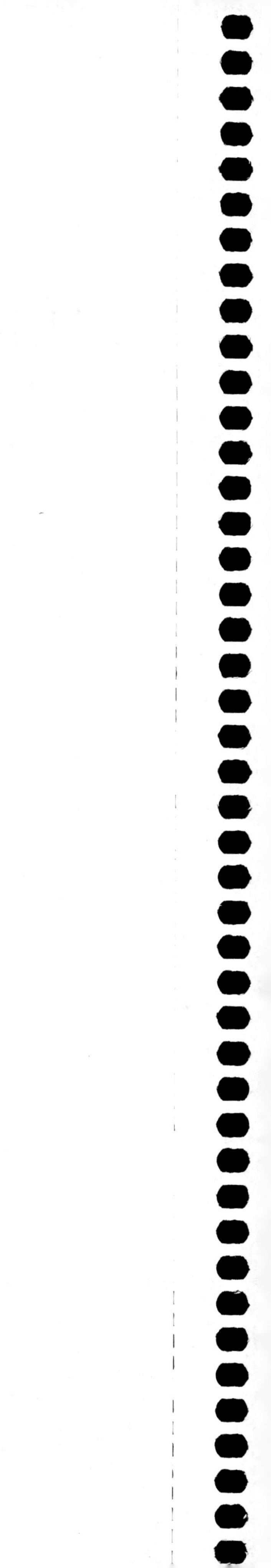

CHAPTER

19

INTERNAL–EXTERNAL MATRIX

The internal–external (I/E) matrix uses the data that was originally assembled in the SWOT analysis (Chapter 9 and Chapter 17) and transferred into the EFE (Chapter 10) and IFE (Chapter 18) analyses, and it helps make sense out of the EFE and IFE results. The I/E matrix positions an organization, or its various divisions, in a nine-cell display, with placement determined by EFE and IFE total scores.

To begin constructing the I/E matrix, the range of possible EFE scores is placed on the vertical axis, and the range of IFE scores is placed in the horizontal axis (see Exhibit 19.1).

The horizontal axis of the matrix reflects internal strength and is divided into three categories: weak (1.0–1.99), average (2.0–2.99), and strong (3.0–4.0). The vertical axis reflects industry attractiveness and is divided into low (1.0–1.99), medium (2.0–2.99), and high (3.0–4.0) categories. The three categories on each axis combine to form nine boxes in the matrix.

The company—or each division, if you have done SWOTs on individual divisions—is then plotted based on the intersection of its IFE and EFE scores. The locations in the I/E matrix correspond to certain standard implied strategies. The strategic groups are marked in Exhibit 19.2 by the letters *A*, *B*, and *C*. The implied strategies corresponding to each letter are listed below the matrix.

Within the I/E matrix, the company or individual divisions are represented as circles. As with the General Electric matrix and the Boston Consulting Group matrix, the sizes of the circles and their pie slices represent the relative significance of each business in terms of sales or profit.

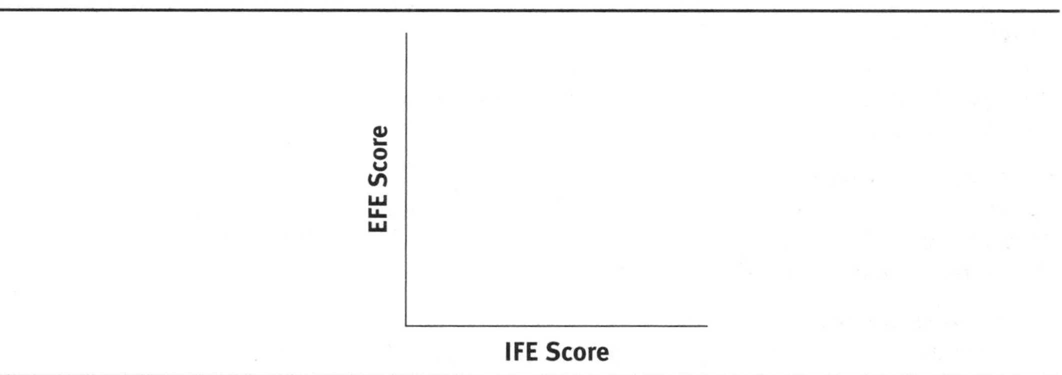

EXHIBIT 19.1
I/E Matrix Construction

EXHIBIT 19.2
I/E Matrix

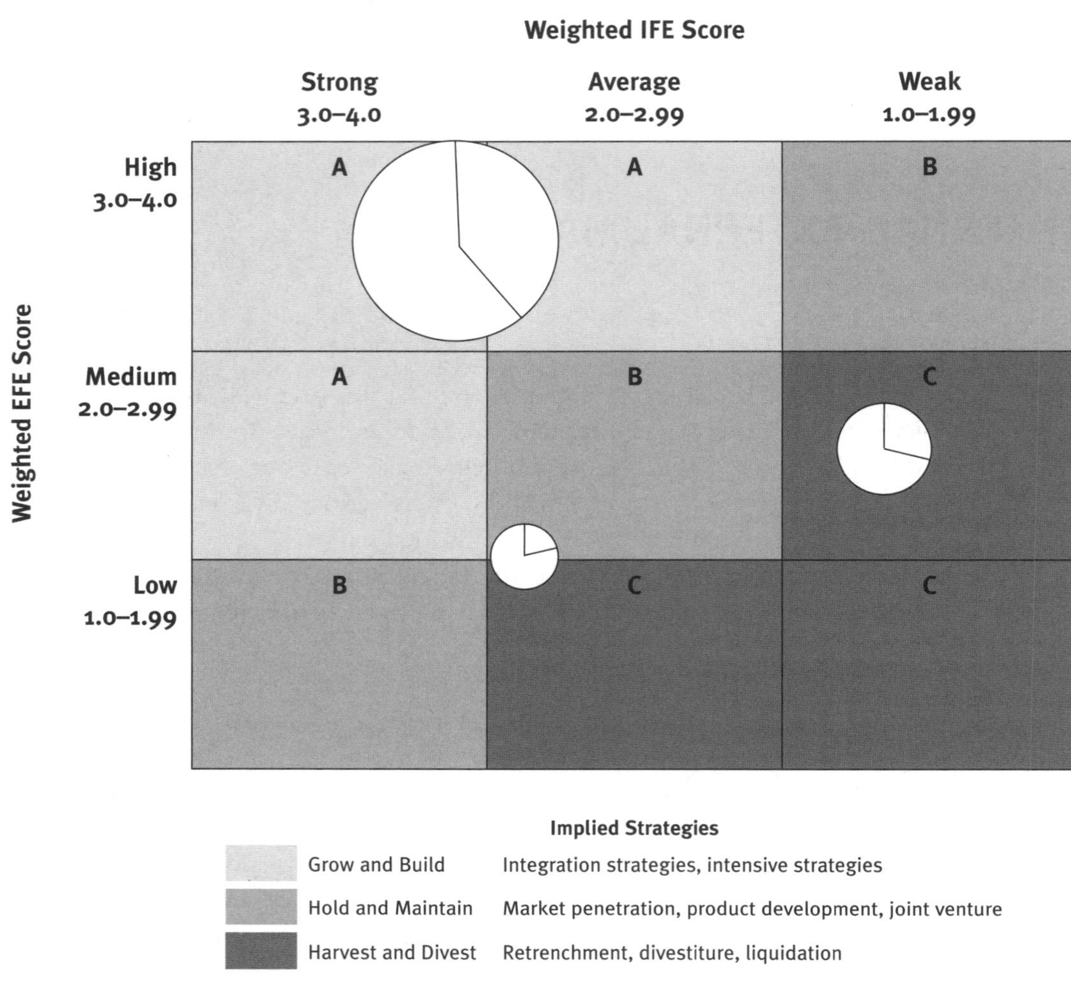

The shaded boxes labeled *A*, *B*, and *C* correspond to certain implied strategies, which are listed in Exhibit 19.2 and more fully explained in Exhibit 19.3. The strategies are broad but are generally considered to be directionally correct.

EXHIBIT 19.3
I/E Matrix Implied Strategies

Integration Strategies
Forward integration: Ownership of or increased control over distributors or retailers
Backward integration: Ownership of or increased control over suppliers
Horizontal integration: Ownership of or increased control over competitors

Intensive Strategies
Market development: Introducing new products or present products into new areas
Product development: Improving or modifying products for increased sales
Market penetration: Increasing share for present products by increased effort

Defensive Strategies
Joint venture: Two or more firms joining and creating a third co-owned firm
Retrenchment: Regrouping via cost- and asset-reduction techniques
Divestiture: Selling a product line, division, or business unit
Liquidation: Selling all company assets

Later, as you begin to develop specific strategies, you can refer back to the I/E matrix and see if your strategy development is consistent with the implied directions. If it is, great! You are on the right path. But if the strategies you are developing are inconsistent with those suggested by the matrix, some serious consideration is needed. For example, if the strategies you develop are all aggressive and the I/ E matrix is suggesting retrenchment or divestiture, a disconnect exists somewhere. The inconsistent strategies do not necessarily have to be abandoned, but they should be closely analyzed. The disconnect may be the result of a weak or improperly constructed analysis. More likely, however, the strategies themselves are inappropriate.

In the space provided, create an I/E matrix for your project organization.

I/E Matrix for ____________________

Weighted IFE Score

Weighted EFE Score	Strong 3.0–4.0	Average 2.0–2.99	Weak 1.0–1.99
High 3.0–4.0	A	A	B
Medium 2.0–2.99	A	B	C
Low 1.0–1.99	B	C	C

Company: ____________________ Scores: __________

Significant issues: ____________________

Division: ____________________ Scores: __________

Significant issues: ____________________

Division: ____________________ Scores: __________

Significant issues: ____________________

Division: ____________________ Scores: __________

Significant issues: ____________________

Division: ____________________ Scores: __________

Significant issues: ____________________

EXERCISE

EXERCISE

Identify the implied strategies. Which make intuitive sense?

1.

2.

3.

4.

5.

CHAPTER

20

GRAND STRATEGY MATRIX

Grand strategies are overarching, long-term strategies that set the direction for a company. The grand strategy matrix (GSM) is intended to assist a strategist in deciding which grand strategies are most appropriate. The GSM is a four-block matrix that considers a company's competitive position in the market as well as the growth rate of the market. These factors are similar to the concepts used in the BCG matrix and the GE matrix.

Any organization can be positioned in one of the GSM's four strategy quadrants. An organization's individual divisions can also be placed in the matrix. To complete a GSM, the analyst identifies whether the company is in a weak competitive position or a strong competitive position. Next, the analyst determines whether the company competes in a market that has rapid growth or slow growth. The intersection of the two positions places the company in one of the four quadrants. Each quadrant lists the appropriate strategies in order of preference for a company in that position (see Exhibit 20.1).

Companies in Quadrant 1 of the GSM are in a great strategic place because they have a strong competitive position in a rapidly growing market. These companies should leverage their existing competitive advantages and focus on their current products and markets. Strategies such as market penetration, market development, and product development are appropriate. If a company in this quadrant has extra cash on hand, it might consider integration strategies such as backward, forward, or horizontal integration. If the company is heavily dependent on a single product or limited customer base, or is in some other way narrowed in scope, concentric diversification may be appropriate.

Companies in Quadrant 2 of the GSM are in a weak competitive position in a growing market. They need to reevaluate their existing strategies to determine why that is. Because the market is growing rapidly, they need to employ intensive strategies such as market penetration, market development, and product development. If a company does not have a tangible competitive advantage, it may try to gain efficiency and economies of scale through horizontal integration. If the strategist believes that a significant competitive advantage cannot be developed and horizontal integration is not an option, the company may choose to sell off the business and use the proceeds from the sale to reinvest in other businesses that may produce a greater return on investment. If a buyer is not available and the company is a cash drain on the parent company, liquidation might be a last resort. In such cases, the company is shut down and its assets are sold to pay debts. Obviously, liquidation is not an attractive strategy, but it could save a parent company from further losses.

Companies in Quadrant 3 have a weak competitive position in a slow growth market. These companies have to take quick action to ensure a turnaround and avoid being driven out of business. Retrenchment tactics, such as cost reductions and sale of assets,

EXHIBIT 20.1
Grand Strategy Matrix

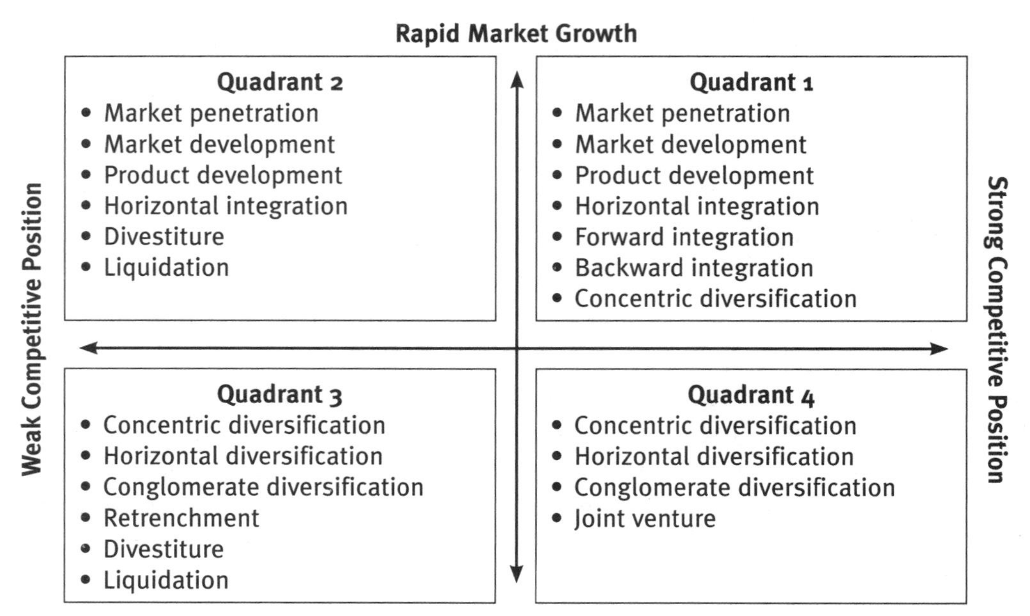

DEFINITIONS

Market penetration: Increasing share for present products by increased effort.
Market development: Introducing new products or existing products into new areas.
Product development: Improving or modifying products for increased sales.
Horizontal integration: Establishing ownership or increased control over competitors.
Forward integration: Establishing ownership or increased control over distributors or retailers.
Backward integration: Establishing ownership or increased control over suppliers.
Concentric diversification: Introducing new products or entering markets related to existing offerings.
Conglomerate diversification: Introducing new products or entering markets unrelated to existing offerings.
Horizontal diversification: Divesting horizontally integrated business units.
Retrenchment: Using cost- and asset-reduction techniques to regroup.
Divestiture: Selling a product line, division, or business unit.
Liquidation: Selling all company assets.

Source: Adapted from Christensen, Berg, and Salter (1976).

can help conserve cash. Alternatively, diversification strategies designed to reposition the business into different areas may be appropriate. These strategies may include horizontal diversification and conglomerate diversification. If all else fails, the company may be sold off or liquidated.

Companies in Quadrant 4 have a strong competitive position but are in a slow growth market. Because of their strength and cash flow, these companies have the ability to reallocate assets into more attractive markets or grow their dominance of the current market. They may pursue these goals through concentric diversification, horizontal diversification, or conglomerate diversification. Additionally, by combining with another company in a strategic joint venture, they can gain further leverage in the market.

Exhibit 20.2 shows a sample GSM for a parent company and three divisions.

EXHIBIT 20.2
GSM Example: Widget, Inc.

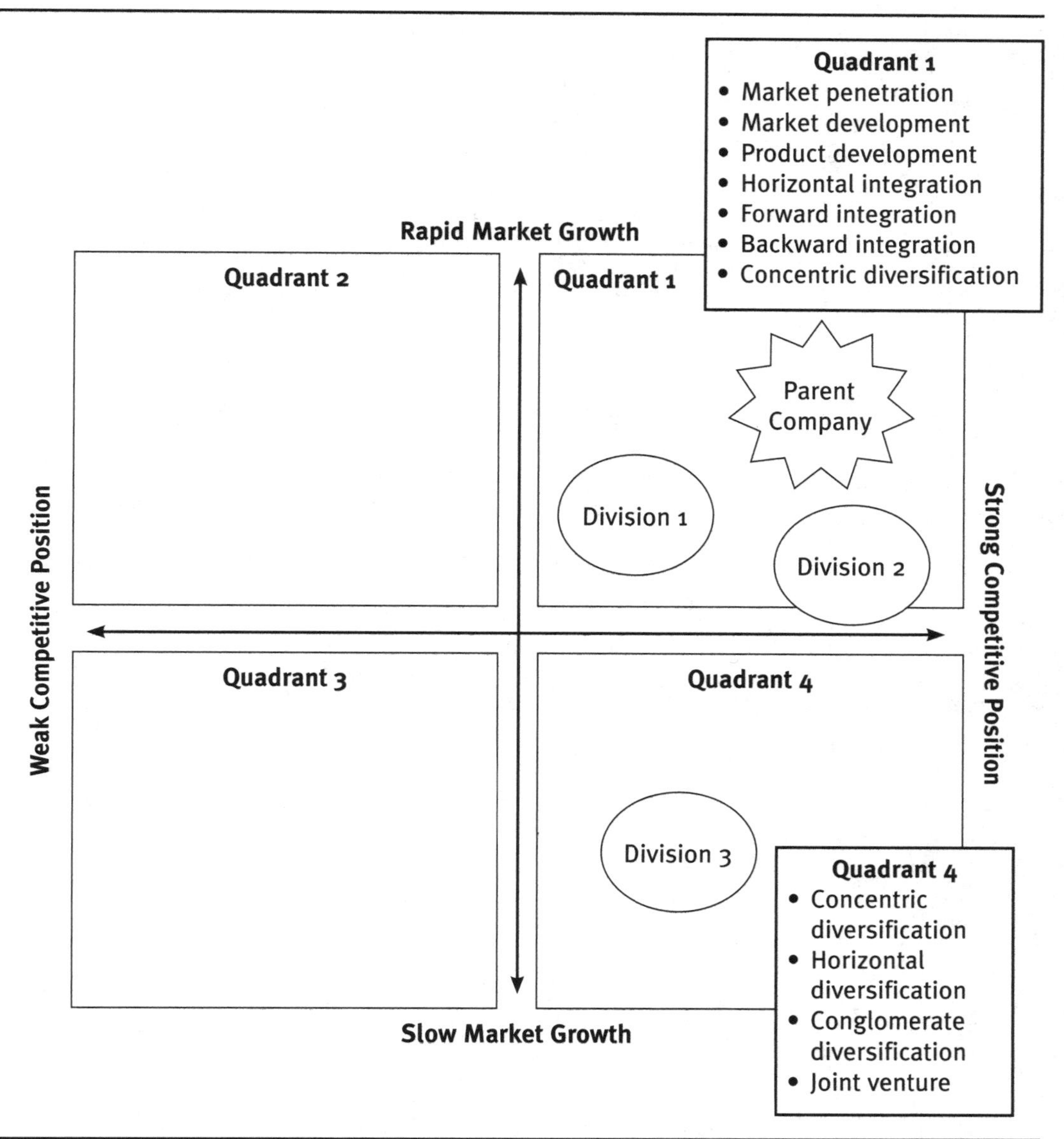

Reference

Christensen, C. R., N. A. Berg, and M. S. Salter. 1976. *Policy Formulation and Administration: A Casebook of Top Management Problems in Business.* Homewood, IL: R. D. Irwin.

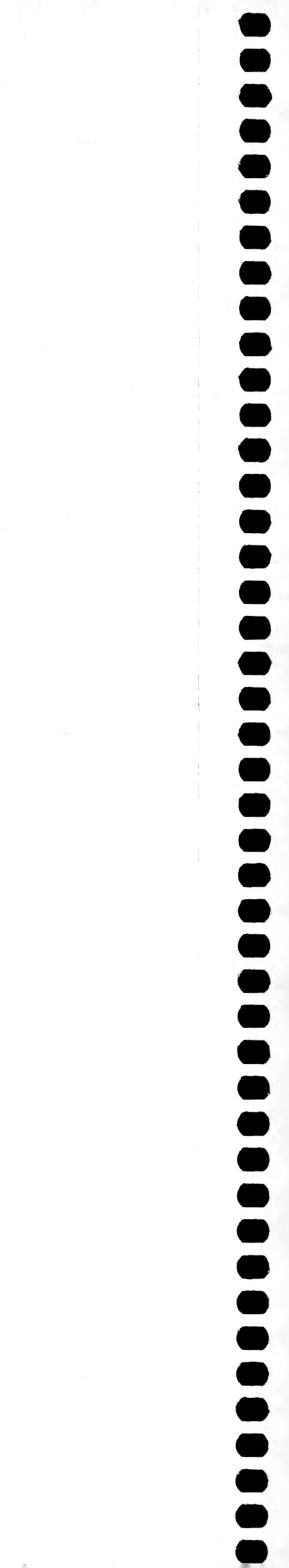

Complete a grand strategy matrix for your project organization.

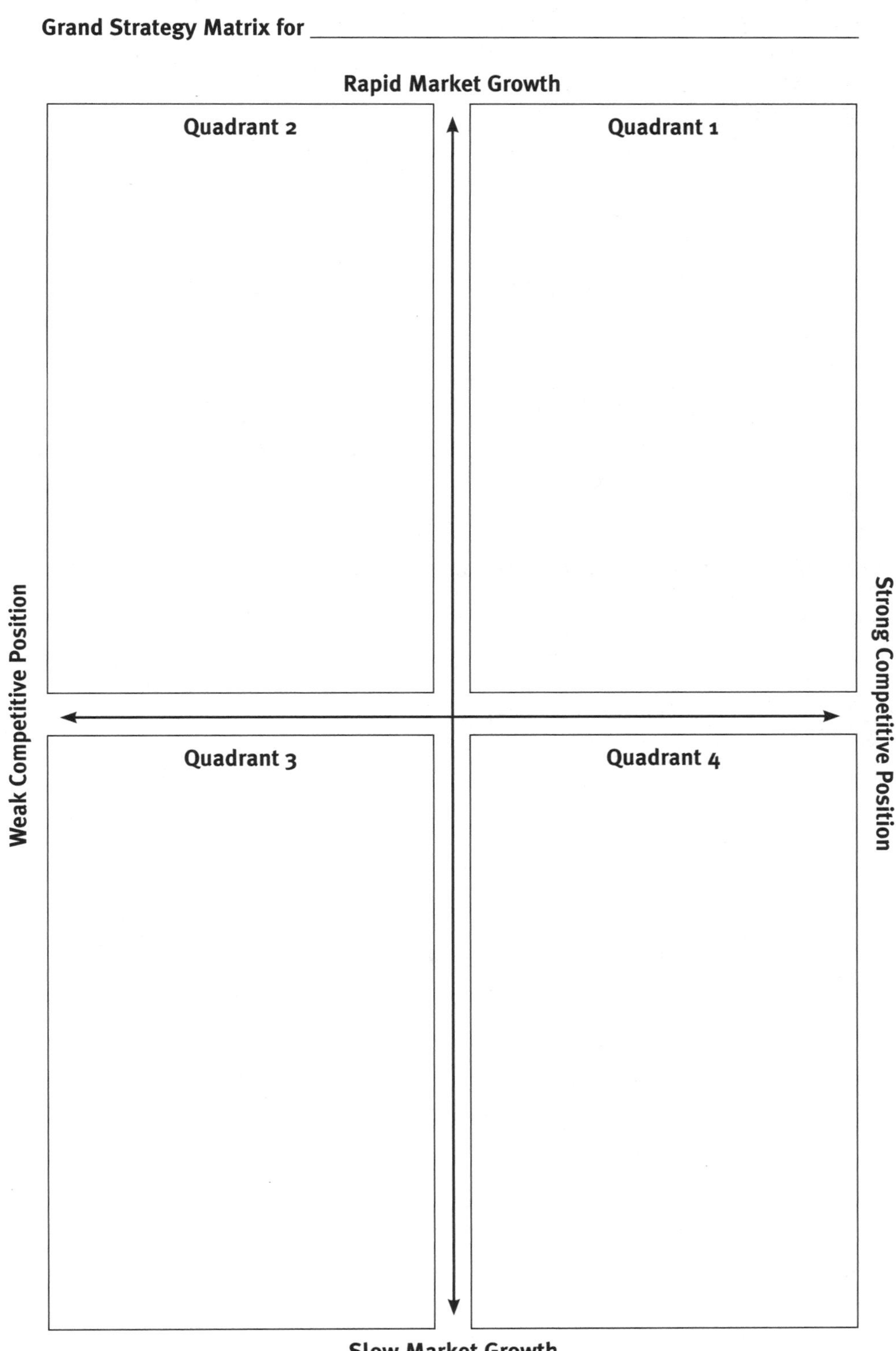

EXERCISE

Explanation:

-
-
-
-
-

Which strategies are appropriate, and which are not? Why?

-
-
-
-
-
-
-

CHAPTER

21 SPACE MATRIX

The strategic position and action evaluation (SPACE) matrix is a four-direction system used to analyze whether conservative, aggressive, defensive, or competitive strategies are most appropriate for a company's approach (Rowe et al. 1982). The analysis looks internally at the company's financial strength and competitive advantage, as well as externally at the stability of the environment and the strength of the industry in which the company competes (see Exhibit 21.1).

In the SPACE matrix, financial strength is plotted against environmental stability, and competitive advantage is plotted against industry strength. Exhibit 21.2 displays the arrangement of the factors on the matrix. A position in the top left quadrant of the SPACE matrix suggests a conservative strategy is appropriate for the company. The top right quadrant suggests an aggressive strategy. The bottom right suggests defensive strategies, and the bottom left suggests competitive strategies.

The steps in completing the SPACE matrix are as follows:

1. Determine what variables to measure. You should have approximately five per factor. The variables should involve critical success factors in the industry and be good indicators of financial strength, competitive advantage, environmental stability, and industry strength. For example, for the issue of financial strength, what are the five or six key indicators of financial health for a company in your industry? Obviously, the variables will change by industry (retail may have very different indicators of financial health than does a hospital), but certain key indicators are common. Some examples are provided below:
   - Financial strength (FS) variables: return on investment (ROI), return on equity (ROE), earnings per share (EPS), leverage, liquidity, other measures from the ratio analysis
   - Competitive advantage (CA) variables: market share, product quality, life cycle position, customer loyalty, manufacturing capability, other factors from the five forces analysis or SWOT
   - Environmental stability (ES) variables: technology, inflation, other factors from PEST and environmental analysis
   - Industry strength (IS) variables: growth potential, profit potential, productivity, other factors from the five forces analysis and environmental analysis

EXHIBIT 21.1
SPACE Matrix Factors

Internal Strategic Position Factors	External Strategic Position Factors
Financial strength (FS)	Environmental stability (ES)
Competitive advantage (CA)	Industry strength (IS)

EXHIBIT 21.2 Elements of a SPACE Matrix

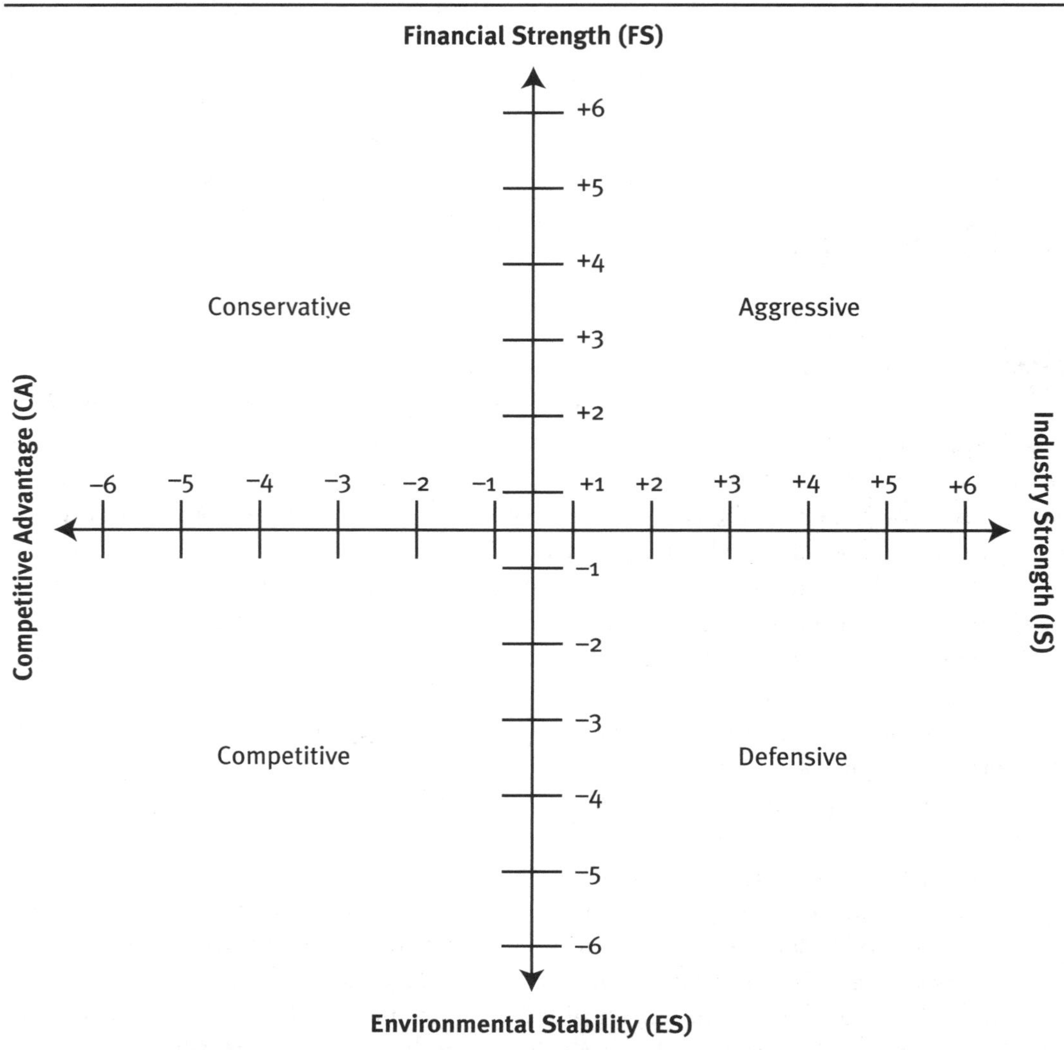

2. Give a score ranging from +1 (terrible) to +6 (great) for each of the variables that make up FS and IS.
3. Give a score ranging from −1 (great) to −6 (terrible) for each of the variables that make up ES and CA.
4. Find the average score for the FS variables, then for the ES variables, then for the CA variables, and finally for the IS variables.
5. Plot the values for each dimension on the appropriate axes of the SPACE matrix.
6. Add the average score for FS to the average score for ES to yield the *y* value.
7. Add the average score for CA to the average score for IS to yield the *x* value. Once you have both an *x* value and a *y* value, you will be able to plot a single point on the SPACE matrix.
8. Find the intersection of the *x*-axis score and the *y*-axis score. Draw a line from the center of the SPACE matrix to the intersection point. This line points to the type of strategies the company should pursue.

Exhibits 21.3 and 21.4 demonstrate the processes of assigning scores for variables, determining *x* and *y* values, and placing your company on the matrix.

EXHIBIT 21.3 Assigning Scores for the SPACE Matrix

	Internal Strategic Position	External Strategic Position
***Y* axis** **Total *y*-axis score:** +4.80 − 2.20 = **+2.60**	**Financial Strength** *(score: +6 best, +1 worst)* +6: EPS increasing +4: Liquidity slightly decreasing +5: ROE increasing +5: ROI increasing +4: Efficiency ratio stable Average: +4.80	**Environmental Stability** *(score: −1 best, −6 worst)* −1: Political elections pending −4: Inflation rate risk −2: Rapid technology change −2: Exchange rates hurting −2: Demographic shifts Average: −2.20
***X* axis** **Total *x*-axis score** −2.40 + 4.60 = **+2.20**	**Competitive Advantage** *(score: −1 best, −6 worst)* −1: Market share −4: New product development −4: Sales force and distribution −1: Patents last 11 more years −2: Human resources and talent development Average: −2.40	**Industry Strength** *(score: +6 best, +1 worst)* +6: Growth potential +5: Barriers to entry +5: Government subsidies +4: Price elasticity +3: Lobbying strength Average: +4.60

EXHIBIT 21.4 Plotting a Company on the SPACE Matrix

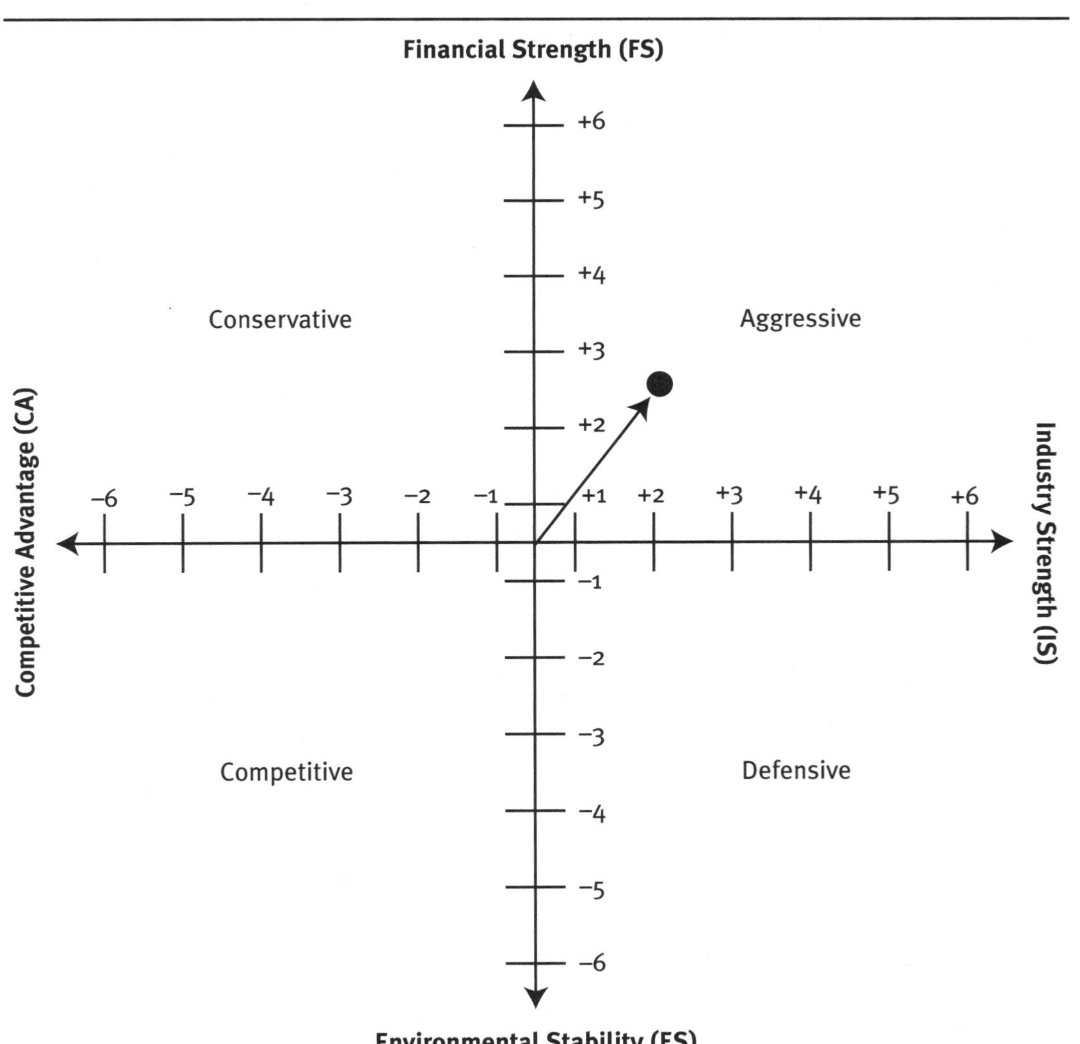

Reference

Rowe, A. J., R. D. Mason, K. E. Dickel, R. B. Mann, and R. J. Mockler. 1982. *Strategic Management and Business Policy: A Methodological Approach.* Reading, MA: Addison-Wesley.

In the space provided, create a SPACE matrix for your project organization.

EXERCISE

SPACE Matrix for ______________________________

	Internal Strategic Position	**External Strategic Position**
***Y* axis** **Total *y*-axis score:** +____ – ____ = [ ]	**Financial Strength** *(score: +6 best, +1 worst)* • • • • • Average: ____________	**Environmental Stability** *(score: –1 best, –6 worst)* • • • • • Average: ____________
***X* axis** **Total *x*-axis score** –____ + ____ = [ ]	**Competitive Advantage** *(score: –1 best, –6 worst)* • • • • • Average: ____________	**Industry Strength** *(score: +6 best, +1 worst)* • • • • • Average: ____________

EXERCISE

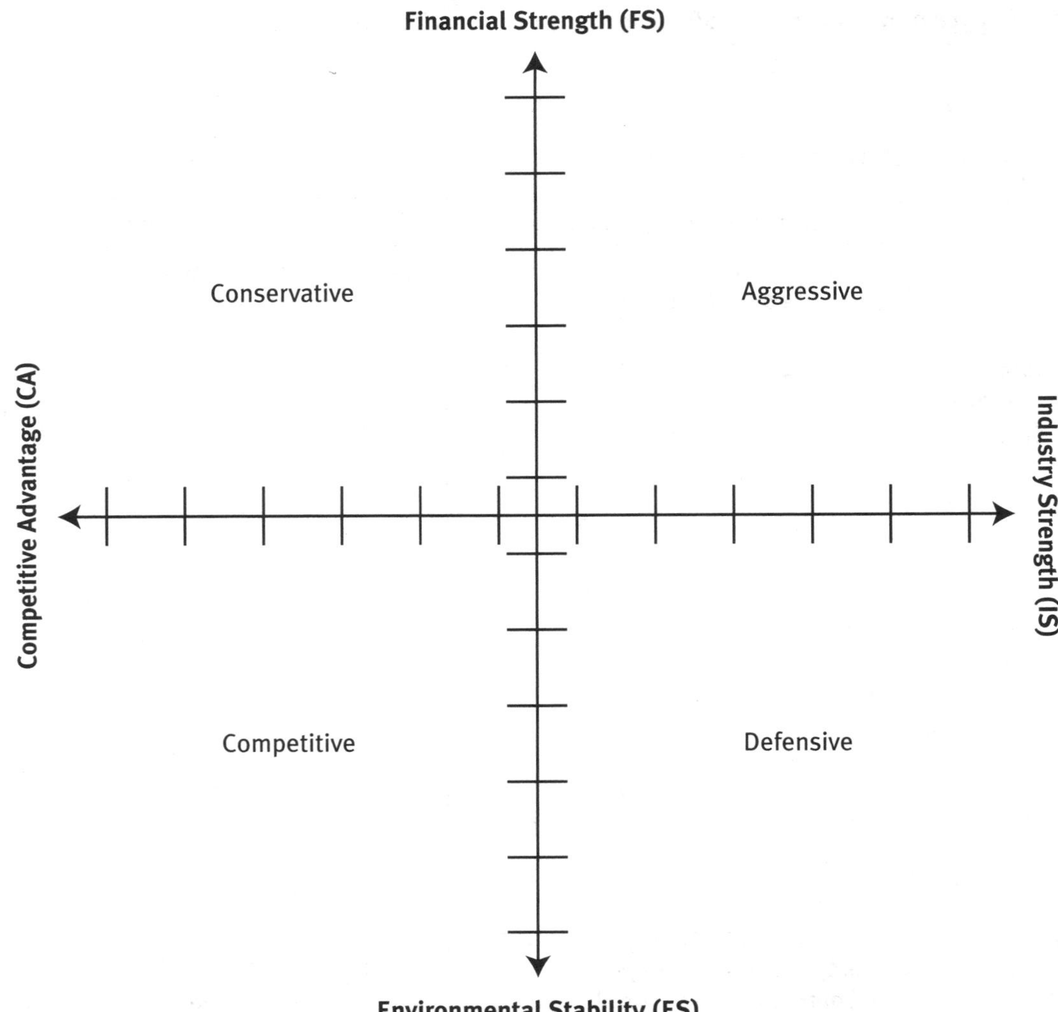
Financial Strength (FS)
Conservative
Aggressive
Competitive Advantage (CA)
Industry Strength (IS)
Competitive
Defensive
Environmental Stability (ES)

PART

V

STRATEGY DEVELOPMENT

CHAPTER 22

GENERIC STRATEGIES

Michael Porter (1980), the originator of the five forces analysis, also identified three general, or generic, strategies that companies can use to compete: cost leadership, differentiation, and focus. These three strategies, displayed in Exhibit 22.1, provide the framework for this chapter.

Cost Leadership Strategy

Cost leadership is a strategy whereby a company chooses to compete in a broad market based on low prices. To compete on price, a company can simply cut its prices, or it can change some other factor in the product, business, or industry. If a company simply cuts price, competitors can do the same thing, and a price war will ensue. In changing some other factor, a company seeks to create a sustainable advantage that does not currently exist. The change may involve the manufacturing process, technology, distribution, process reengineering, cost cutting, or any other area that affects the cost side of the equation for the company. A reduction on that side of the equation can be passed on to buyers of the product or service in the form of lower prices.

A lower price for a comparable product is expected to undercut the competition and drive up sales and market share. For example, many companies have sought to lower their costs by outsourcing business processes to other countries where certain tasks can be

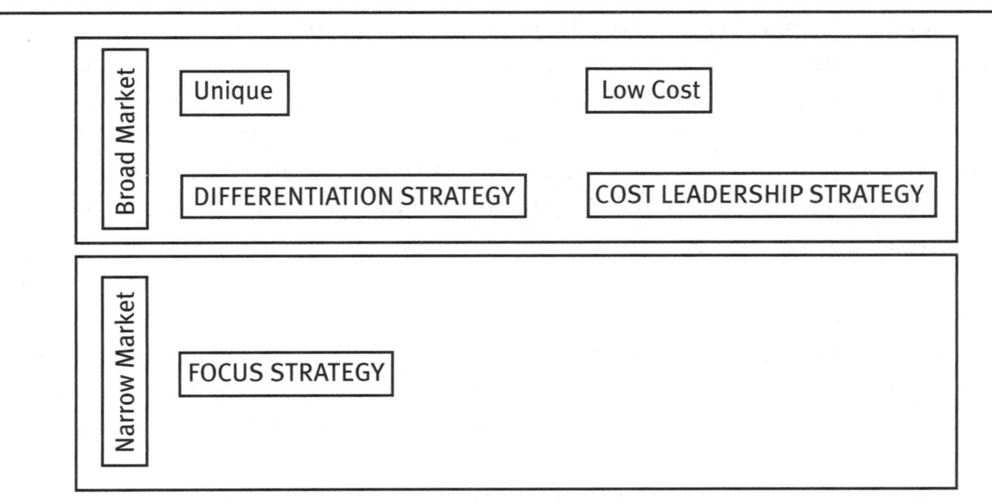

EXHIBIT 22.1 Generic Strategies Compared to Market and Approach

completed more cheaply. Sometimes, a company will simplify a product and offer a "no-frills" version that can be produced in high volume with low cost. Some large companies (e.g., Wal-Mart) may leverage their size and scope to squeeze lower prices from their suppliers. Maintaining a low-cost strategy requires a company to constantly search for new ways to cut costs and increase efficiency, because competitors will likely seek to replicate any advantage.

Wal-Mart and others that use cost leadership strategies are now deeply involved in healthcare, with walk-in clinics, low-cost pharmacies, and optical and other services. This trend is expected to continue as the emphasis on cost reduction intensifies across the industry. The Affordable Care Act (ACA) is a major driver of this cost reduction, and organizations that use cost leadership as their strategic approach may be well positioned for the future of healthcare delivery.

Differentiation Strategy

Differentiation involves creating a product or service that is perceived as superior or unique by the buyer in the broad market. To the extent that the buyer believes that a product is unique and that the uniqueness is valuable, the buyer will be willing to pay a higher price. Thus, companies may compete on the uniqueness of products rather than on price. Often, buyers will develop brand loyalty and continue to purchase the same product over time, even if they have to pay a slight premium (e.g., BMW cars). The difficulty is that the perceived exclusivity of a product can make it harder to mass market, and the higher cost associated with differentiating the product's features can drive up price.

In healthcare, providers and hospitals alike try to differentiate themselves in a variety of ways. For instance, many organizations use the latest in technology to attract patients who are seeking healthcare services. Others use marketing campaigns to inform consumers of specialty credentials.

Focus Strategy

A focus strategy centers on a particular niche, customer type, product line segment, or geography. By segmenting the market and choosing to focus on one or two specific segments, a company can tailor its offering to the specific needs and desires of the target. By better serving the target, the company can maintain higher profit margins. Sometimes start-up companies use a focus strategy to gain a foothold and then later shift to other strategies to broaden their market. The trade-off with the focus strategy is often high profit margin versus low sales volume, and vice versa.

Numerous examples of this strategic approach can be seen in healthcare. A high degree of specialization exists among healthcare providers, and this trend is due in part to the low reimbursement levels for primary care providers in comparison to specialists. The ACA has aimed to address the need for more primary care providers by increasing reimbursement for their services, and we are now seeing more mid-level practitioners assuming those roles.

Generally, companies compete using only one strategy for a product rather than combining strategies. Maintaining a "low-cost/high-volume" strategy at the same time as a "differentiation/premium-price" strategy, for instance, is difficult. The exception to this rule is that a focus strategy can sometimes be combined with a component of the other two strategies. For example, a focus strategy might add a low-price component to target a niche market, although the low profit margin and small market would be difficult in the long term. Likewise, a focus strategy might add a differentiation component, although the small market combined with the higher cost of a differentiated product could also be untenable in the long run.

Reference

Porter, M. E. 1980. *Competitive Strategy: Techniques for Analyzing Industries and Competitors.* New York: Free Press.

CHAPTER

23

ANSOFF MATRIX

The Ansoff matrix is an analytical tool used to assist a company in developing its product and market growth strategies. The matrix was first published in the *Harvard Business Review* in 1957. It is sometimes called the product/market expansion grid (Ansoff 1957).

The Ansoff matrix can be used to categorize an existing strategy, to determine the risk associated with a new or proposed strategy, or to develop new strategies. For our purposes, we will focus on the matrix as a strategy development tool. The matrix considers products or services in comparison to the markets the company proposes to serve. The matrix compares these factors on the basis of whether each is new or existing. Markets are placed on the vertical axis, and products and services are placed on the horizontal axis. The intersection of these axes creates four possible blocks (see Exhibit 23.1).

The bottom left box represents strategies aiming to provide existing products to existing markets. Such strategies are considered "market penetration" because they involve driving existing products deeper into existing markets. A company's efforts in this area may seek to attract new customers, but they are still within the same overall market. Market penetration is the least risky box on the grid: The company already knows its products, services, and customers.

The top left box represents strategies aiming to provide existing products to new markets. Strategies of this type are considered "market development" because they involve driving existing products into markets that are currently unserved by the organization. For example, consider a local eye care provider that seeks to enter a market it has not served previously with products and services (Lasik surgery, for instance) that are new to that market. Due diligence indicates that the market has a need for the service, but the provider must repackage its marketing materials and other aspects of its business to meet the needs of the new market. Developing a new market for an existing service or product is a moderate-risk proposition: The provider knows its product well but is entering an unknown market.

EXHIBIT 23.1
Ansoff Matrix

MARKETS		Existing	New
	New	**Market Development** *(Risk = moderate)*	**Diversification** *(Risk = high)*
	Existing	**Market Penetration** *(Risk = low)*	**Product Development** *(Risk = moderate)*

PRODUCTS AND SERVICES

The bottom right box—labeled "product development"—involves developing new products for existing markets. A company typically knows its market and patients/customers well, and it may have insights as to what the market's unmet needs are. The company may then create new products or services to meet these needs. Continuing the above example of the eye care organization, the company could attempt to provide optical services or contact lenses for the market it has entered. These services would be different from the Lasik surgery the organization already offers, but they could serve the same market and meet the market's needs. Developing a new product for an existing market is a moderate-risk proposition: The company knows its customers well but is developing an unknown product.

The top right box—"diversification"—is the box with the highest risk, because the company is creating new products for new markets. It is essentially approaching a double unknown. Perhaps our eye care provider brings in hearing services. The transition introduces new patients/customers and a completely new service and product. Even if the organization has experience with hearing services in other locations and finds them to be a successful adjunct to its eye care services and products, this is nonetheless a high-risk strategy.

To use the Ansoff matrix, lay out the four-box grid format and brainstorm specific strategies that correspond to each box. For example, begin with new products for existing customers. What are the needs of your existing market and customers? Try to identify at least five unmet needs and five potential approaches to address these needs. Repeat this process for the remaining three boxes. If you successfully brainstorm a large number of ideas, pick the top five for inclusion in the matrix.

Reference

Ansoff, I. 1957. "Strategies for Diversification." *Harvard Business Review* 35 (5): 113–24.

In the space provided, create an Ansoff matrix for your project organization.

EXERCISE

Ansoff Matrix for ______________________________

MARKETS	Existing (Products and Services)	New (Products and Services)
New	Market Development *(Risk = moderate)* 1. 2. 3. 4. 5.	Diversification *(Risk = high)* 1. 2. 3. 4. 5.
Existing	Market Penetration *(Risk = low)* 1. 2. 3. 4. 5.	Product Development *(Risk = moderate)* 1. 2. 3. 4. 5.

PRODUCTS AND SERVICES

CHAPTER

24

TOWS STRATEGY DEVELOPMENT

The TOWS matrix is one of the most widely used strategy development tools. It adapts the SWOT matrix (see Chapters 9 and 17) to develop specific strategic options for your company. Under TOWS, the SWOT components are matched in pairs, and strategies are developed to address them. When matched, the SWOT factors yield four groups of strategic options (Weihrich 1982).

To construct the TOWS matrix, boxes for the SWOT components are placed on the outside of a four-cell matrix, with strengths and weaknesses on the horizontal axis and opportunities and threats on the vertical axis. Exhibit 24.1 demonstrates the construction.

The intersections of the SWOT components form the basis of the TOWS strategy pairs, which occupy the four matrix boxes as shown in Exhibit 24.2. The TOWS pairs are named according to the initials of the intersecting components—SO, WO, ST, and WT. The strategic approaches suggested by each pair are explained in Exhibit 24.3.

Unlike the previous matrices we have looked at, the TOWS matrix is used to develop specific, rather than generic, strategies. The matrix uses SWOT for the format and draws upon all the previous analyses and matrices to develop a knowledge base from which specific strategies are created.

EXHIBIT 24.1
Construction of a TOWS Matrix

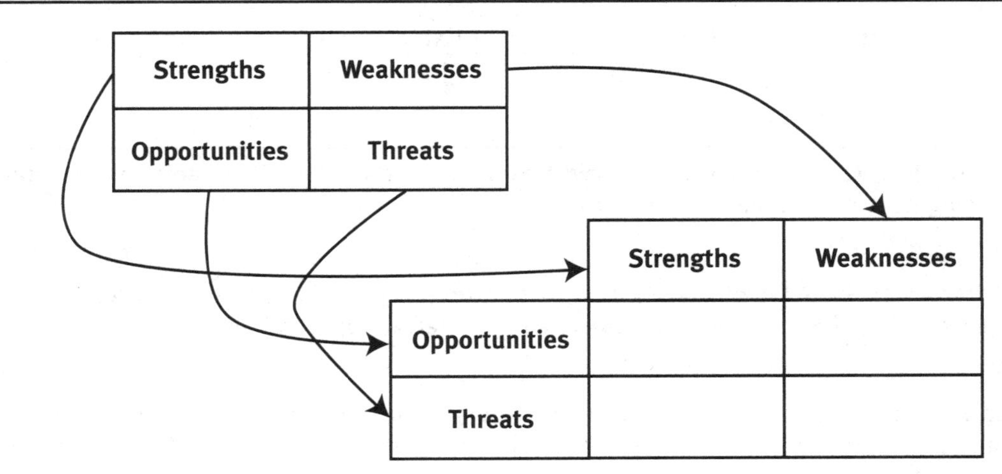

EXHIBIT 24.2
TOWS Strategy Pairs

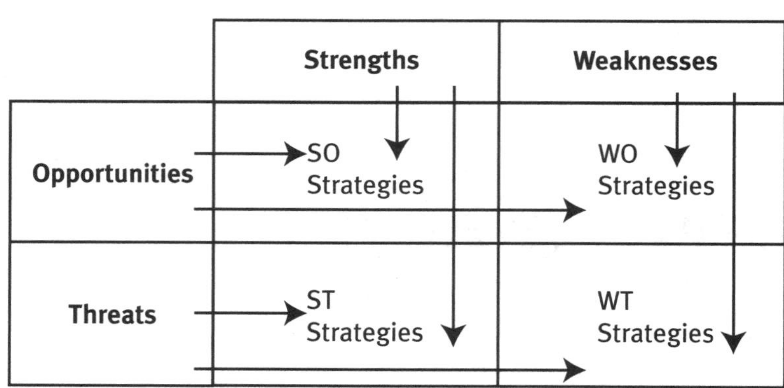

To develop specific strategies, the strategist lists all the SWOT items in each SWOT box. Then the strategist looks at the intersections of the boxes and attempts to match SWOT issues and develop specific strategies to address matched pairs. For example, if a strength was listed as, "The company has strong cash flow with significant cash on hand," and an opportunity was listed as, "Numerous competitors are available for sale," then a potential SO strategy might be, "Leverage the company's strong cash position (S) to horizontally integrate by buying competitor Acme (O)."

After each strategy, the specific SWOT pair from which the strategy is derived is identified inside parentheses. For example, if a particular strategy addresses the fifth strength and the seventh opportunity, it would be identified as "Strategy (S5, O7)."

The strategist should attempt to develop five to ten feasible or potential strategies per block. Not all strategies will be viable, but they should be reasonable. You are not necessarily endorsing or keeping the strategies just because you list them here. Specific strategy selection will come later. The task here is to come up with as many reasonable alternatives as possible. TOWS development is best done by team brainstorming in order to capitalize on each team member's strengths and differing thought processes.

The partially completed TOWS matrix in Exhibit 24.4 builds on the example from earlier chapters about SWOT analysis.

EXHIBIT 24.3
Definitions of TOWS Pairs

SO strategies: Match internal strengths with external opportunities. These strategies leverage the strengths to exploit the opportunities.

WO strategies: Match internal weaknesses with external opportunities. These strategies compensate for internal weaknesses by exploiting external opportunities.

ST strategies: Match internal strengths with external threats. These strategies attempt to use strengths to avoid or reduce the impact of external threats.

WT strategies: Match internal weaknesses with external threats. These strategies are defensive in nature and attempt to reduce internal weaknesses and avoid external threats. Generally, these strategies do not create strengths but rather protect from loss.

EXHIBIT 24.4
TOWS Example

	Strengths	**Weaknesses**
	1. Local market dominance 2. Caring staff 3. Excellent administration 4. Good location 5. Outstanding facilities 6. Strong community support 7. Excellent board of trustees 8. Expanding to meet growth 9. Center of regional healthcare 10. Technology	1. Weak process to manage low-income population 2. Inability to manage population without health coverage 3. No process to address transient market 4. Difficulty recruiting providers 5. Reputation of the facility 6. Not addressing changes in reimbursement 7. Staff turnover 8. Nursing shortage 9. Need for technical staff 10. Limited resources in mental health
Opportunities 1. Expansion of existing services 2. Additional locations 3. Greater exposure and branding 4. Addition of trauma center 5. Purchasing additional practices 6. Expansion into surrounding counties 7. Government contracts 8. Residency programs/teaching 9. Expansion of ancillary services 10. Demographic changes	**SO Strategies** 1. Use local market dominance to expand into urgent care (S1, O1). 2. Leverage the existing good location to place new satellite locations (S4, O2). 3. 4. 5.	**WO Strategies** 1. Use residency programs and teaching to overcome difficulty recruiting providers (W4, O8). 2. Leverage opportunity to open new locations to attract nurses (W8, O2). 3. 4. 5.
Threats 1. Multiple competitors 2. Emergency department overcrowding 3. Power of suppliers 4. Recent lawsuits 5. Low socioeconomic status 6. Transient market 7. Dependence on suppliers 8. Difficulty recruiting providers 9. Changes in reimbursement 10. Decrease in population	**ST Strategies** 1. Use organizational expansion to overcome power of suppliers (S8, T3). 2. Use the excellent administration to overcome difficulty recruiting providers (S3, T8). 3. 4. 5.	**WT Strategies** 1. Settle recent lawsuits in order to improve the reputation of the facility (W5, T4). 2. Become expert at reimbursement process in order to overcome changes in reimbursement levels (W6, T9). 3. 4. 5.

Reference

Weihrich, H. 1982. "The TOWS Matrix—A Tool for Situational Analysis." *Long Range Planning* 15 (2): 54–66.

In the space provided, create a TOWS matrix for your project organization.

TOWS Matrix for ______________________________

	Strengths	**Weaknesses**
	1. 2. 3. 4. 5. 6. 7. 8. 9. 10.	1. 2. 3. 4. 5. 6. 7. 8. 9. 10.
Opportunities 1. 2. 3. 4. 5. 6. 7. 8. 9. 10.	**SO Strategies** 1. 2. 3. 4. 5. 6. 7. 8. 9. 10.	**WO Strategies** 1. 2. 3. 4. 5. 6. 7. 8. 9. 10.
Threats 1. 2. 3. 4. 5. 6. 7. 8. 9. 10.	**ST Strategies** 1. 2. 3. 4. 5. 6. 7. 8. 9. 10.	**WT Strategies** 1. 2. 3. 4. 5. 6. 7. 8. 9. 10.

EXERCISE

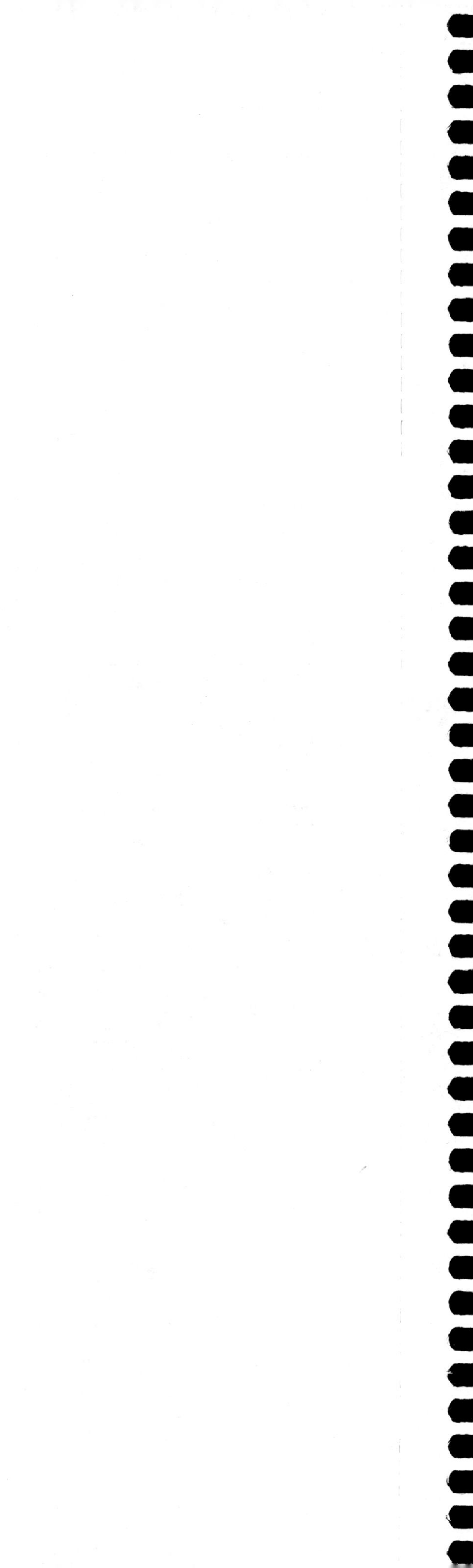

PART

VI

STRATEGY SELECTION

CHAPTER

25 STRATEGIC FIT AND THE QUANTITATIVE STRATEGIC PLANNING MATRIX

To begin the process of strategy selection, the analyst reviews the potential strategies identified in the Ansoff and TOWS matrices. Many strategists place each possible strategy on a separate sticky note, so the strategies can be sorted and moved around into clusters. The strategist searches for commonalities among the strategies. Most likely, about 25 strategies can be grouped under four or five main headings. The strategist identifies those main headings and places the appropriate strategies under each. The main headings become "overarching strategies," and the specific strategies from the Ansoff and TOWS matrices become "supporting strategies" or "substrategies."

Exhibit 25.1 provides an example of strategy consolidation from the Ansoff and TOWS matrices. "Expand into adjacent counties," "Expand into urgent care," "Place satellite locations," "Open cancer center," and "Buy out private practices" could all be grouped under the overarching strategy of "facility expansion." Likewise, many Ansoff and TOWS example strategies could be consolidated under the overarching strategy of "service expansion."

Pursuing every good strategy is not recommended. An organization likely will not have sufficient funds to pursue every option, and doing so would lead to a lack of focus. The strategic options need to be culled and the most promising ones retained.

After the strategies have been consolidated, the analyst can evaluate the strategies at two levels. First, the overarching strategies can be compared against one another. For

EXHIBIT 25.1 Strategy Consolidation

Facility Expansion	Consolidated from Ansoff and TOWS matrices	Service Expansion
1. Expand into adjacent counties.		1.
2. Expand into urgent care.		2.
3. Place satellite locations.		3.
4. Open cancer center.		4.
5. Buy out private practices.		5.

example, in Exhibit 25.1, facility expansion would be compared with service expansion. At the second level, the substrategies under an overarching strategy can be evaluated and then either retained or discarded. In the facility expansion example, the analyst would decide whether to retain or discard "Expand into adjacent counties," "Expand into urgent care," "Place satellite locations," "Open cancer center," and "Buy out private practices."

Strategic Fit Assessment

To choose among the overarching strategies, the strategist constructs a quantitative strategic planning matrix (QSPM) (David 1986). This matrix assesses each overarching strategy based on how attractive it is relative to the external factor evaluation (EFE) and internal factor evaluation (IFE) factors (see Chapters 10 and 18). This assessment produces an attractiveness score (AS) and a total attractiveness score (TAS) for each strategy. The strategy with the highest total attractiveness score is the strategy considered most appropriate for implementation.

To create the QSPM, place the external opportunities and threats from the EFE analysis and the internal strengths and weaknesses from the IFE analysis into the left column of the matrix. Make sure you list at least ten external factors and ten internal factors. Include the weight from the IFE and EFE with each item.

The attractiveness score in the QSPM indicates whether each IFE/EFE factor is important to, has a significant impact on, or produces an "attractive" match with each strategy. The scores are determined by analyzing each IFE/EFE factor and considering whether the factor makes a difference in the decision of which strategy to pursue. If the factor does not make a difference, the attractiveness score is zero. If the factor does make a difference, the strategy is rated relative to that factor. The rating scale, from 0 to 4, is shown in Exhibit 25.2.

Once the attractiveness scores have been assigned, each factor's score for each strategy is multiplied by the weight associated with that factor. The product of each multiplication is the total attractiveness score for each factor.

Exhibit 25.3 shows a QSPM for two strategies being evaluated head to head. Note that any number of strategies can be compared to one another using the QSPM. We have presented just two in Exhibit 25.3 for ease of explanation. The more likely scenario is that a strategic analyst will compare between two and five viable strategies.

To more closely examine the QSPM example, we will focus on a specific external opportunity, "Greater exposure and branding," shown in Exhibit 25.4. To assign numbers to this row, the analyst must consider the two strategies against the opportunity of gaining more exposure and branding. The opportunity's weight of 0.050 comes from the EFE matrix.

EXHIBIT 25.2
Attractiveness Rating Scale

1 = not attractive
2 = somewhat attractive
3 = reasonably attractive
4 = highly attractive
0 = not applicable

EXHIBIT 25.3
QSPM Example

			Facility Expansion		Service Expansion	
		Weight	Attractiveness Score	Total Attractiveness Score	Attractiveness Score	Total Attractiveness Score
Opportunities						
1.	Expansion of existing services	0.050	3	0.150	4	0.200
2.	Additional locations	0.100	4	0.400	4	0.400
3.	Greater exposure and branding	0.050	4	0.200	3	0.150
4.	Addition of trauma center	0.025	4	0.100	4	0.100
5.	Purchasing additional practices	0.025	3	0.075	3	0.075
6.	Expansion into surrounding counties	0.075	4	0.300	4	0.300
7.	Government contracts	0.025	1	0.025	2	0.050
8.	Residency programs/ teaching	0.025	2	0.050	1	0.025
9.	Expansion of ancillary services	0.050	1	0.050	4	0.200
10.	Demographic changes	0.050	1	0.050	2	0.100
Threats						
1.	Multiple competitors	0.100	2	0.200	2	0.200
2.	Emergency department overcrowding	0.100	4	0.400	2	0.200
3.	Power of suppliers	0.025	2	0.050	2	0.050
4.	Recent lawsuits	0.025	0	0.000	0	0.000
5.	Low socioeconomic status	0.050	2	0.100	2	0.100
6.	Transient market	0.075	3	0.225	1	0.075
7.	Dependence on suppliers	0.025	1	0.025	1	0.025
8.	Difficulty recruiting providers	0.075	2	0.150	1	0.075
9.	Changes in reimbursement	0.025	3	0.075	0	0.000
10.	Decrease in population	0.025	2	0.05	1	0.025
	Total weight:	1.000				
Strengths						
1.	Local market dominance	0.100	3	0.300	2	0.200
2.	Caring staff	0.050	2	0.100	2	0.100
3.	Excellent administration	0.050	3	0.150	2	0.100
4.	Good location	0.025	3	0.075	3	0.075
5.	Outstanding facilities	0.050	3	0.150	2	0.100
6.	Strong community support	0.025	3	0.075	3	0.075

(continued)

EXHIBIT 25.3
QSPM Example (continued)

			Facility Expansion		Service Expansion	
		Weight	Attractiveness Score	Total Attractiveness Score	Attractiveness Score	Total Attractiveness Score
7.	Excellent board of trustees	0.025	2	0.050	2	0.050
8.	Expanding to meet growth	0.050	4	0.200	3	0.150
9.	Center of regional healthcare	0.050	3	0.150	2	0.100
10.	Technology	0.075	2	0.150	1	0.075
Weaknesses						
1.	Weak process to manage low-income population	0.050	1	0.050	1	0.050
2.	Inability to manage population without health coverage	0.100	1	0.100	1	0.100
3.	No process to address transient market	0.025	1	0.025	1	0.025
4.	Difficulty recruiting providers	0.025	2	0.050	3	0.075
5.	Reputation of the facility	0.050	2	0.100	3	0.150
6.	Not addressing changes in reimbursement	0.100	1	0.100	1	0.100
7.	Staff turnover	0.050	2	0.100	2	0.100
8.	Nursing shortage	0.025	2	0.050	2	0.050
9.	Need for technical staff	0.025	1	0.025	2	0.050
10.	Limited resources in mental health	0.050	1	0.050	2	0.100
	Total weight:	1.000		4.725		4.175

For facility expansion, the analyst has assigned an attractiveness rating of 4, meaning that the strategy is highly attractive for the exposure and branding opportunity. The AS of 4 is multiplied by the weight of 0.050 to arrive at a TAS of 0.200. Next, the strategy of service expansion is rated the same way. The analyst in the example has given the strategy a score of 3 relative to the factor of gaining more exposure and branding. The 3 is multiplied by the weight of 0.050 for a TAS of 0.150. Comparing the TAS of each strategy, one can see that facility expansion is the more favorable strategy relative to the opportunity (0.200 versus 0.150).

EXHIBIT 25.4
Specific Factor Example

			Facility Expansion		Service Expansion	
		Weight	Attractiveness Score	Total Attractiveness Score	Attractiveness Score	Total Attractiveness Score
3.	Greater exposure and branding	0.050	4	0.200	3	0.150

When all the IFE/EFE factors have been assigned scores, the TAS column for each strategy is summed. This process yields a total score for each strategy relative to all the factors. The bottom row of Exhibit 25.3 shows that, considering all the EFE/IFE factors, the facility expansion strategy is quantitatively more attractive than the service expansion strategy (4.725 versus 4.175).

The quality of the QSPM, as with all the matrices, depends on the quality of the work put in by the analyst. Although the matrix is quantitative by nature, the assignment of scores, the choice of internal and external factors, and the weights are all subjective. The analyst must do a thorough job in each of the previous matrices and fully understand the organization and its market. Intuition and human decisions remain imperative even in a quantitative model.

Assessing the Supporting Strategies

The supporting strategies within the overarching strategy can be assessed next. Not all the supporting strategies will be appropriate, and some may be mutually exclusive. Many strategists run a QSPM again on the supporting strategies and retain those with the highest scores. Other analysts use research and intuition to determine which ones stay and which go. The cost of implementing one supporting strategy might affect how many other strategies the company can afford to take on. At the same time, multiple supporting strategies might be necessary for successful completion of the overarching strategy.

Consistency Check

Once strategies have been selected, they should be checked for consistency with the directional matrices discussed in previous chapters. If the grand strategy matrix, SPACE matrix, and internal–external (I/E) matrix suggest a conservative strategy and the strategist has chosen an aggressive overarching strategy with aggressive supporting strategies, then something is wrong. The inputs and decision making may need to be reconsidered.

Reference

David, F. R. 1986. "The Strategic Planning Matrix—A Quantitative Approach." *Long Range Planning* 19 (5): 102–7.

EXERCISE

In the space provided, draft a QSPM for your project organization.

QSPM for ________________

Opportunities	Weight	Strategy 1		Strategy 2		Strategy 3		Strategy 4	
		Attractiveness Score	Total Attractiveness Score	Attractiveness Score	Total Attractiveness Score	Attractiveness Score	Total Attractiveness Score	Attractiveness Score	Total Attractiveness Score
1.									
2.									
3.									
4.									
5.									
6.									
7.									
8.									
9.									
10.									

(continued)

EXERCISE

Threats	Weight	Strategy 1		Strategy 2		Strategy 3		Strategy 4	
		Attractiveness Score	Total Attractiveness Score	Attractiveness Score	Total Attractiveness Score	Attractiveness Score	Total Attractiveness Score	Attractiveness Score	Total Attractiveness Score
1.									
2.									
3.									
4.									
5.									
6.									
7.									
8.									
9.									
10.									
Total weight:									

EXERCISE

			Strategy 1		Strategy 2		Strategy 3		Strategy 4	
		Weight	Attractiveness Score	Total Attractiveness Score	Attractiveness Score	Total Attractiveness Score	Attractiveness Score	Total Attractiveness Score	Attractiveness Score	Total Attractiveness Score
Strengths										
1.										
2.										
3.										
4.										
5.										
6.										
7.										
8.										
9.										
10.										

(continued)

EXERCISE

Weaknesses	Weight	Strategy 1		Strategy 2		Strategy 3		Strategy 4	
		Attractiveness Score	Total Attractiveness Score	Attractiveness Score	Total Attractiveness Score	Attractiveness Score	Total Attractiveness Score	Attractiveness Score	Total Attractiveness Score
1.									
2.									
3.									
4.									
5.									
6.									
7.									
8.									
9.									
10.									
Total weight:		TAS:		TAS:		TAS:		TAS:	

CHAPTER

26

FINANCIAL FIT ASSESSMENT AND PROJECTION

In strategy selection, the financial investment required to support implementation is a significant criterion, as is the amount of time needed to recoup the investment and profit potential. The QSPM model might show one proposal to be superior to the others in a strategic sense; however, the organization might not have the financial resources to successfully implement and maintain that strategy. To address concerns of this nature, the strategist must apply a financial screen to the proposed strategies.

In a survey of 1,139 executives by McKinsey & Company, 75 percent said companies that get the best results use a balanced mix of financial and strategic targets; only 11 percent disagreed (Dye, Sibony, and Truong 2009). The point behind these findings is that a strategic fit is not enough. One needs both a strategic fit and a financial fit.

A complete financial analysis, using factors such as depreciation, tax effect, and so on, is beyond the scope of this book. However, this chapter introduces several important financial analysis measures, including net present value, internal rate of return, profitability index, payback period, and probability of success.

Net Present Value

The net present value (NPV) of a future stream of income recognizes that the future income is worth less in today's dollars than a simple arithmetic sum of the same dollars would indicate. The basic idea behind this concept is that a dollar in hand today is worth

EXHIBIT 26.1
Example of Net Present Value

Data	Description
10%	Annual discount rate
\$(10,000,000)	Initial cost of investment one year from today
\$3,000,000	Return (less costs) from first year
\$4,200,000	Return (less costs) from second year
\$6,800,000	Return (less costs) from third year
\$4,000,000	Total return
\$1,188,443	**NPV**

Excel syntax: NPV(rate,value1,value2, . . .)

more than the promise of a dollar five years from now. The promise five years from now will be eaten away by inflation, which lessens the dollar's purchasing power.

Exhibit 26.1 demonstrates a calculation for net present value using Microsoft Excel. To begin, set up a chart showing the annual cost of capital or discount rate, followed by each yearly income. You can then use Excel's "=NPV" function to calculate the net present value. Use the discount rate as "rate," and highlight the cells with the initial cost and yearly incomes to finish the equation. In the example shown in the exhibit, the total return less the up-front investment is $4,000,000; however, the net present value is only $1,188,443 due to the time value of money.

Internal Rate of Return

The internal rate of return (IRR) determines the percentage return on an investment considering an initial start-up expenditure followed by an annual income stream. The measure enables a strategist to compare one strategy to another to determine which has the highest percentage return. Some companies use the discount rate for comparison with the IRR. However, most companies have a discreet decision criteria threshold such as, "Any project investment must have an IRR of 10 percent or greater, or we will not pursue it."

Exhibit 26.2 shows a Microsoft Excel calculation of internal rate of return. Using the same chart you used for calculating the NPV, select Excel's "=IRR" function and then highlight the cell with the initial cost plus the cells with the yearly incomes to finish the equation. Excel allows a space in the syntax for "guess," but we recommend that you leave this field blank, in which case Excel will automatically assume 10 percent. In the example shown in the exhibit, the total income less the up-front investment is $4,000,000, and the internal rate of return is 16 percent.

Profitability Index

The profitability index (PI) is similar to the internal rate of return, but it is calculated differently and gives a slightly different percentage return. The PI provides information on your strategic investment opportunity, as well as a decision rule by which you can

EXHIBIT 26.2
Example of Internal Rate of Return

Data	Description
10%	Annual discount rate
$(10,000,000)	Initial cost of investment one year from today
$3,000,000	Return (less costs) from first year
$4,200,000	Return (less costs) from second year
$6,800,000	Return (less costs) from third year
$4,000,000	Total return
16%	**IRR**

Excel syntax: IRR(value1,value2, . . ., Guess)

EXHIBIT 26.3
Example of Profitability Index

Data	Description
10%	Annual discount rate
$(10,000,000)	Initial cost of investment one year from today
$3,000,000	Return (less costs) from first year
$4,200,000	Return (less costs) from second year
$6,800,000	Return (less costs) from third year
$4,000,000	Total return
$1,188,443	NPV
1.12	**PI**

Formula: (NPV + start-up costs) / start-up costs
($1,188,443 + $10,000,000) / $10,000,000

accept or reject an investment. The PI tells you what your return will be for every dollar invested in a strategic initiative (e.g., for every $1 invested you will return $1.29). The PI also suggests that a project with a PI score of less than 1 should be rejected as an insufficient return, whereas a project with a PI score of 1 or greater should be considered for investment.

Exhibit 26.3 adds profitability index to our previous example. Because the PI in the example is greater than 1, the standard rule suggests the project should be considered and not rejected. For every $1 invested in this strategy, the total value created is $1.12—a 12 percent return.

Payback Period

The payback period (PP) answers the question, "If I make the required investment in this strategy, how long will it take to recoup my investment?" This period can be expressed in the number of months or number of years. In the previous example, the payback period is approximately 30 months to recoup the initial $10,000,000 invested (excluding the time value of money).

Probability of Success

Potential strategies will each have different likelihoods of success, and a strategy's profit potential should be discounted by the probability of achieving it. You can estimate the probability of success based on research and intuition, and then multiply the probability by the NPV. This calculation enables you to compare across potential strategies that have different NPVs and different probabilities of success, to level the comparison playing field.

EXHIBIT 26.4 Comparison of Values

	NPV	IRR	PI	PP	Prob	Prob*NPV	Choice
Strategy A	$28.1M	15.1%	1.2	7.1yrs	91%	$26.133M	1st
Strategy B	$30.7M	16.3%	1.3	7.5yrs	85%	$24.867M	2nd

Putting It Together

Lining up the various calculations in a single display, as shown in Exhibit 26.4, allows you and your viewer to quickly see the values and thus more easily compare competing strategies to find the best financial fit with your company. Keep in mind that a strategy with a good financial fit might not be a good strategic fit; likewise, a strategy with a great strategic fit might not make the most financial sense.

Final Thoughts

Strategy is important, and it can provide an organization with a significant competitive advantage and the ability to meet the challenges of tomorrow. Some may say that you can't predict what the future holds, but remember the old adage: Failure to plan is planning to fail! It is the sincere belief of the authors that this workbook provides you and your organization with the tools you need to meet the challenges of the rapidly evolving healthcare marketplace. Only through effective strategic management will you be able to maintain and grow your market position in this dynamic environment.

Thank you for using this book, and best wishes for a successful future!

Reference

Dye, R., O. Sibony, and V. Truong. 2009. "Flaws in Strategic Decision Making: McKinsey Global Survey Results." *McKinsey Quarterly*. Published January. www.mckinsey.com/insights/strategy/flaws_in_strategic_decision_making_mckinsey_global_survey_results.

GLOSSARY OF STRATEGIC ANALYSIS TERMS

affinity chart: A method of organizing ideas generated in brainstorming and arranging the ideas under conceptual headings. See Chapter 2.

Ansoff matrix: An analytical tool that considers products or services in comparison to the markets the company proposes to serve. The matrix compares these factors on the basis of whether each is new or existing. The four blocks in the matrix represent different strategies. See Chapter 23.

Boston Consulting Group (BCG) matrix: An approach to strategic analysis that compares a firm's market share to the anticipated growth of its market. The quadrants of the matrix place organizations into four categories: "stars," "question marks," "cash cows," and "dogs." See Chapter 12.

brainstorming: A process for generating ideas in a group setting where individuals feel free to voice opinions and share suggestions. See Chapter 2.

competitive market benchmark analysis: A method for understanding the position of competitors in the market and using comparisons and differentiation to drive strategy development. See Chapter 8.

cost leadership strategy: A strategy whereby a company chooses to compete in a broad market based on low prices. See Chapter 22.

differentiation strategy: A strategy based on creating a product or service that is perceived as superior or unique by the buyer in the broad market. See Chapter 22.

external factor evaluation (EFE): A system for organizing and evaluating opportunities and threats—the external aspects of SWOT. The EFE produces a score that reflects the gravity of each issue combined with management's current response to it. See Chapter 10.

financial ratio analysis: An approach that combines internal analysis of an organization's finances with external comparisons, using financial ratios from various categories. See Chapter 11.

five forces analysis: An approach for analyzing industry factors that are likely to affect strategy. The five forces are threat of entry, intensity of rivalry, threat of substitute products, bargaining power of suppliers, and bargaining power of buyers. See Chapter 6.

focus strategy: A strategy that centers on a particular niche, customer type, product line segment, or geography. See Chapter 22.

future-perfect thinking: A planning tool that involves projecting oneself into the future, determining what the perfect future situation would be, and then imagining how it occurred. See Chapter 2.

General Electric (GE) matrix: A nine-block business screen in which a business's overall strength is compared to the overall attractiveness of the market within which the business competes. See Chapter 13.

grand strategy matrix (GSM): A four-block matrix that considers a company's competitive position in the market (strong or weak) and the growth rate of the market (rapid or slow). Each quadrant lists appropriate strategies. See Chapter 20.

internal–external (I/E) matrix: A nine-cell display in which an organization is placed based on its internal factor evaluation (IFE) and external factor evaluation (EFE) scores. The nine cells correspond with certain implied strategies. See Chapter 19.

internal factor evaluation (IFE): A system for organizing and evaluating strengths and weaknesses—the internal aspects of SWOT. The IFE produces a score that reflects the gravity of each issue. See Chapter 18.

internal rate of return (IRR): A measure of the percentage return on an investment considering an initial start-up expenditure followed by an annual income stream. See Chapter 26.

life cycle analysis: An approach that assesses organizations based on the current stage in their life cycle. Researchers have generally identified five main phases in a life cycle: birth, growth, maturity, revival, and decline. See Chapter 15.

McKinsey 7S model: A framework for organizational effectiveness that focuses on seven components—strategy, structure, systems, staff, skills, style, and shared values—and emphasizes coordination among them. See Chapter 14.

mission statement: The expression of an organization's pure mission (what we do), vision (where we are going), and values (how we will get there). See Chapter 4.

net present value (NPV): A measure of the current value of a future stream of income, accounting for the time value of money. See Chapter 26.

organizational culture analysis: Study of the system of shared values, meanings, and beliefs that influences the way an organization's members act toward one another. See Chapter 16.

payback period (PP): The amount of time needed to recoup the money invested in a project. See Chapter 26.

PEST analysis: A process for examining the environment through political, economic, social, and technological perspectives. See Chapter 7.

profitability index (PI): A measure that provides information on the expected return on an investment opportunity, as well as a decision rule by which you can accept or reject an investment. See Chapter 26.

quantitative strategic planning matrix (QSPM): A tool for assessing strategies based on how attractive they are relative to the external factor evaluation (EFE) and internal factor evaluation (IFE) factors. The matrix produces scores for each strategy being compared. The strategy with the highest total attractiveness score is the one considered most appropriate for implementation. See Chapter 25.

strategic industry map: A matrix that provides a "snapshot" of an entire industry. Typically, one axis has some combination of price/quality/image, and the other has a measure of product mix. See Chapter 5.

strategic position and action evaluation (SPACE) matrix: A four-direction system for analyzing whether conservative, aggressive, defensive, or competitive strategies are most appropriate for a company. The analysis looks internally at the company's financial strength and competitive advantage and externally at the stability of the environment and the strength of the industry. See Chapter 21.

SWOT analysis: A method for examining an organization's strengths, weaknesses, opportunities, and threats. Strengths and weaknesses are considered internal aspects of SWOT; opportunities and threats are external aspects. See Chapters 9 and 17.

TOWS matrix: An adaptation of the SWOT analysis that develops specific strategic options. The SWOT components (strengths, weaknesses, opportunities, and threats) are matched in pairs, yielding four groups of strategic options (SO, WO, ST, and WT). See Chapter 24.

About the Authors

Michael S. Wayland is assistant professor of management at Methodist University in Fayetteville, North Carolina, where he has taught business policy and strategy since 2007. Prior to joining Methodist, he worked in various management positions for Fortune 500 companies such as Chrysler Motors, PepsiCo, and General Electric. He received his undergraduate degree from Providence College and his master's degree from Wayne State University.

Warren G. McDonald, PhD, is professor and chair of the Department of Health Care Administration at Methodist University. He is also chief executive officer of McDonald and Associates, LLC, a healthcare consulting firm. His academic background includes undergraduate degrees in opticianry and management, graduate degrees in healthcare management (Norwich University) and education (East Carolina University), and a doctor of philosophy degree in health sciences (Touro University), along with a number of professional certifications. He is a member of the class of 2005 at the Institute for Management and Leadership in Higher Education at Harvard University, and he holds a graduate certificate in healthcare risk management from the University of Florida. He is a noted lecturer at conferences across the country and abroad.